# *3000 Shoes from 1896*

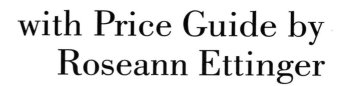

with Price Guide by
Roseann Ettinger

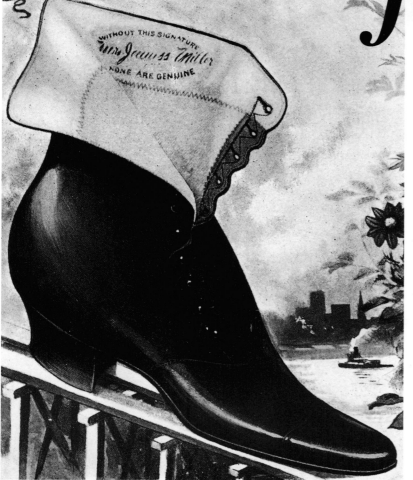

WITHOUT THIS SIGNATURE

NONE ARE GENUINE

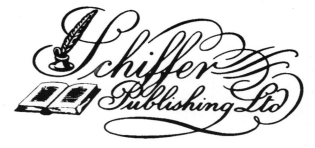

Schiffer Publishing Ltd

4880 Lower Valley Road, Atglen, PA 19310   USA

CW00644443

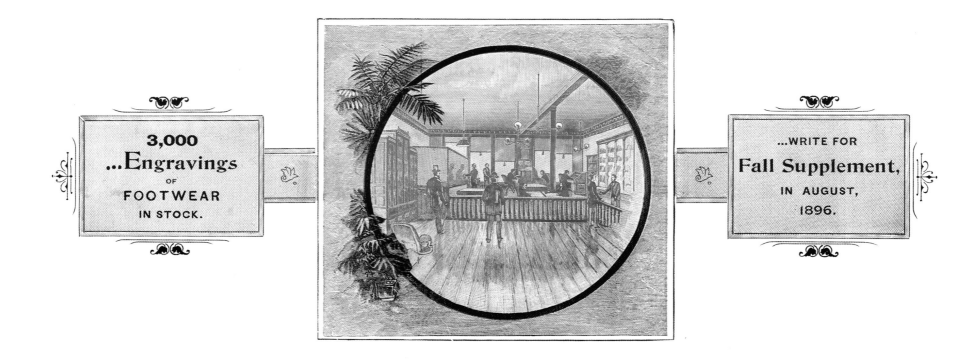

**3,000 ...Engravings** OF **FOOTWEAR** IN STOCK.

...WRITE FOR **Fall Supplement,** IN AUGUST, 1896.

Cover: Advertisment for The Jenness Miller Hygienic Shoe for Women manufactured by Dalton Shoe Company, Dalton, Massachusetts, 1898.

Copyright © 1998 by Roseann Ettinger
Library of Congress Catalog Card Number: 98-84542

Designed by "Sue"
Type set in Bodoni Bd Bt/Bodoni Bk Bt

ISBN: 0-7643-0606-5
Printed in China.

Published by Schiffer Publishing Ltd.
4880 Lower Valley Road
Atglen, PA 19310
Phone: (610) 593-1777; Fax: (610) 593-2002
E-mail: Schifferbk@aol.com
Please write for a free catalog.
This book may be purchased from the publisher.
Please include $3.95 for shipping.

In Europe, Schiffer books are distributed by
Bushwood Books
6 Marksbury Avenue
Kew Gardens
Surrey TW9 4JF England
Phone: 44(0)181-392-8585; Fax: 44(0) 181-392-9876
E-mail: Bushwd@aol.com

Please try your bookstore first.

We are interested in hearing from authors
with book ideas on related subjects.

# 3,000 ENGRAVINGS

## OF FOOTWEAR

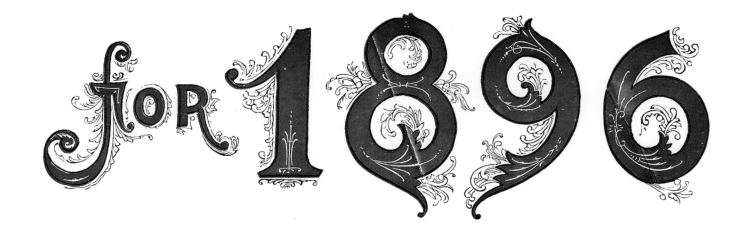

# for 1896

FOR SALE BY

# GEO. D. RAMSDELL,

## ROCHESTER, N.Y., U.S.A.

## "JENNESS MILLER" HYGIENIC SHOES FOR WOMEN!

## DALTON SHOE CO. DALTON, MASS.

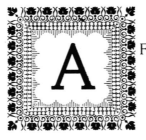

AFTER nearly two years of phenomenal success under the most severe test at the National Capital, the "Jenness Miller" Hygienic Shoes have been perfected and are now ready to be placed on the market. Their success in Washington, where they were controlled by Mr. F. Crocker, has been phenomenal, and he to-day is in daily receipt of mail orders for the "Jenness Miller" Shoes throughout the United States. Testimonials have been received from every State in the Union commending the "Jenness Miller" Shoes for their unequaled comfort, elegance, style and durability. The hygienic anatomical principle upon which these shoes are built is the product of the fertile brain of Mrs. Jenness Miller, an interview with whom appears on another page. These shoes are an entirely different last from any now on the market, and are made in "welts" and "turns," button and lace, in the "common-sense" and narrower "dress" lasts. They are also made in Oxfords. Each pair is stamped with the fac-simile autograph of Mrs. Jenness Miller on top facing and sole.

They are made from "VELVETTA" kid, which is tanned expressly for the "Jenness Miller" Shoe, and is controlled by us, and is as soft and fine as its name implies. They are as comfortable and as durable as modern skill and ingenuity can make them.

The "Jenness Miller" Shoes will be confined to one leading dealer in each city in America under contract to maintain their standard retail price of $3.50 and $5.00. This gives the dealer the advantage of a staple, permanent, never-changing style, and thus eliminates all losses through "clearance" sales and ruinous price-cutting. You pay no more for the famous "Jenness Miller" Shoes than for any other high-grade shoe made to retail at $3.50 and $5.00. The manufacturers also contract with the dealer to advertise the "Jenness Miller" Shoe extensively, both nationally and in the leading local newspapers over the signature of the local merchant. Applications for the exclusive agency for the famous "Jenness Miller" Hygienic Shoes should be made at once.

# A LETTER TO YOU.

THIS book is not late as you may think if you will consider the amount of labor it has taken to make it. It is a study to keep posted with the various styles of shoes that are up to date, therefore a book of this kind takes time when so many styles are illustrated. Now here is nearly 3,000 designs for you to select from. It would cost you $18,000 to get these cuts made to order, it cost me $1,500 to print and mail it. I expect to get it back by selling some of these stock cuts. Do not think that because I can make an electrotype or a duplicate for 20 cents, that I can afford to print this book and find you and give you discounts, etc., etc. Of course there are a great many cuts that may never sell, but nobody knows what somebody else wants. A great many of these circulars are sent abroad, therefore you should not be concerned with some of these cuts that are of later date. I have made hundreds of different styles that are not illustrated in this book, and the reason I have not got them, is because I could not get permission to use them, nor could I bargain for them. How do I get these cuts? Answer—Nine-tenths of them I make up by grading for this book only, and again, I get a great many by making exchanges with my customers. I paid $237.00 to one of my customers for the privilege of using the children's spring heels on two pages of this book. I offer no cuts for sale in stock that do not belong to me, or that I have no right to sell, still many of them are very similar with but slight changes from those I have made for others. I intend to issue a supplement for fall styles, and for 1897, just as soon as the styles can be had, but cannot tell just when. If you are a customer of mine you will receive it without the asking, if you are not on my books, then you will have to send for it. If you have any use for this book I advise you to save it, as the lot is apt to run out, and I shall never print another of this size.

---

## LOOK AT THAT CUT ☞

### It is a ZINC ETCHED PLATE.

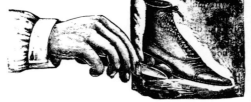

I WARN YOU to beware of some concerns that are trying to catch your trade by showing you samples of shoes of which they generally appropriate (or steal) the outlines from my shoes, then make in this way and by calling the process unknown, etc. It is made on a ZINC ETCHED PLATE. The paper it is drawn on is white enamel cardboard, then printed jet black on the surface. It is then stamped or embossed, as you see in the illustration, the knife scrapes off the black showing the white dots, then a ZINC PLATE is made from this scratch drawing, and if printed on nice plate paper direct from the original plate the result is quite attractive, but if you take an electrotype of it and print on cheap paper you will find the job no good at any price. Beware of half-tone, wax, and all other processes. They fill up in printing, therefore you do not want them.

Very truly yours,

GEO. D. RAMSDELL.

THE CUTS IN THIS SUPPLEMENT ARE FOR SALE TO ALL

# Shoe Dealers, Manufacturers, Wholesalers and Jobbers,

But not to any concern that will or intends to duplicate them or resell them in any such way as I offer in this book. Any concern found copying or offering for sale any parts of these illustrations will be prosecuted for infringing on my copyright.

BEWARE of Concerns in Chicago and elsewhere that show you prints of shoes that are mostly copied from my outlines. Their drawings are made on SCRATCH PAPER with a knife (see illustration) to imitate Halftone engraving, then ZINC plates are etched. Plates are no good, and not deep, the electrotypes too shallow to print on plain paper. Beware! you do not want them at any price.

IF YOU HAVE NOT MY BACK CATALOGUES PRINTED IN 1892, 1893 and 1894, SEND 6 CTS. IN STAMPS FOR THEM. THEY HAVE OVER 1,200 SHOE CUTS OF BACK STYLES, AND SOME 40 PICTURE CUTS FOR ADVERTISING. I ALSO HAVE SOME 20 LARGE SHOE CUTS FOR STREET CAR ADVERTISING.

THESE STOCK CUTS WERE ALL ENGRAVED ON WOOD, the lines are cut extra deep and as coarse as is necessary for all kinds of press printing—such as Catalogue and Newspaper work. *What you buy will be called Duplicates or Electrotypes,* they have a copper face and are blocked on wood, type high, unless you order metal base, which will cost you one-third more. For instance, an electrotype mounted on wood that costs 20 cents, would cost 30 cents mounted on metal. There is no use in having them mounted on metal, and they are too heavy to ship by mail.

TIME. I always keep a few extra electros and can fill small orders immediately, but when the names are ordered engraved on the side of shoes it takes one day longer to make extra electrotypes. Parties who intend to order more electros from a cut they have ordered their name engraved on, can *leave their original cut with me,* to order extra electros from *in the future.* This will save time *and the expense* of re-engraving the name and buying the cut again.

PRICES. The prices for stock cuts in this book will be found at the bottom of each page. On all orders of $25.00 or more, 5 per cent. discount ; $100.00, 10 per cent. discount. This applies to Stock Cuts only. Any order of $5.00 or less, with CASH enclosed, I will mail free of charge. *Make out your order* according to prices in this book, stating Number of shoe at the left, the price to the right. *Do not cut them out.* Do not lose time in asking for discounts, these are the only prices I will make. With good reference I give 30 days' time.

The prices in this book are for Stock Cuts only, and apply to only one order, unless your original is left with me to hold for your future orders, as above stated.

CHANGES. REMEMBER, I will PUT IN OR TAKE OUT TIPS on any shoe free of charge. Send a pencil sketch or pattern of the tip you want, or mention some other number that has the tip you want. I will also remove space stitch lines, and change military heels to opera heels, heel foxes, tops, and bend toes down or up on side view shoes.

NAMES. I charge $1.00 *to engrave a name* on the side of a shoe *in a relief letter* (that means a black letter in a white place). 50 cents where it can be cut in white letters *on a black place.*

CHANGES. When you order changes on a shoe that you pay $1.00 for, or on a front toe that you pay 50 cts. for, no extra charges for the change. You can then have extra electros made at 20 cts. each from the one that is changed, but I will not make changes on a shoe if the shoe wanted can be found in this book, nor will I change one shoe more than once at one price. This means if you get more than one style out of one shoe you will be charged Stock Cut prices for each style.

ORDER BY NUMBERS—*Do not cut them out.*

HOW TO ORDER. To a few people who do not quite understand my prices, the following bill will explain :

| | |
|---|---:|
| Send us Stock Cut of shoe No. 1188 | $1.00 |
| Put our name on the side of same | 1.00 |
| Put on Front View Tip No. 1203 on same block | .50 |
| Also Sole No. 833 | .50 |
| And 20 extra electros of Shoe, Sole and Tip on same block, at 30c. | 6.00 |
| | $9.00 |

*Please hold Originals for future orders.*

Enclosed find draft for the same on New York, Boston or Philadelphia.

Ship per American Express.

MANUFACTURERS can use these cuts for any advertising purpose they like, such as Catalogues and Newspaper advertising.

MORE CUTS. I will have a supplement about the first of August and November, 1896. These will only be sent to parties who ask for them.

PRICES TO MANUFACTURERS FOR NEW OR ORIGINAL CUTS FROM THEIR SHOES.

MANUFACTURERS should order side view shoe cuts with front view tips attached to same cut for illustrating catalogues ; this illustrates the whole shoe and does not take up extra space in printing, and when extra electrotypes are ordered with tips attached to shoe cuts, there is no extra charge for the electrotype of the tip as there is on soles. *In ordering new cuts* from your shoes send me the shoe you want, one shoe only of each style, say the right foot shoe ; size 3 is the best. Write on a slip of paper the number of shoe, style of view, front toe, sole, and what name is wanted on the side, how many electros, etc. ; put the slip in the shoe and send to me by express. I do not care for the last in the shoe.

I charge manufacturers $5.00 each for original shoe cuts, with their name engraved on the side, cuts 2⅛ inches right to left, and $2.50 each for soles with the name or stamp ; $2 without the stamp on sole, and $2 each for front view tips. Extra electrotypes of a shoe of this size, 20 cents each ; of a shoe and sole on one block, 30 cents each ; all low shoes with sole, 25 cents each ; of a sole separate from the shoe, 20 cents each ; of a front view toe separate from shoe, 20 cents each ; when front view toes are ordered with the shoe on same block, no extra charge for the electrotyping of front toe. On all orders of $50 or more, when given at one time, 5 per cent. discount. Terms, 30 days with good reference.

These are my prices to all manufacturers for designing and engraving original shoes. I am the only Designer and Engraver in the United States that makes a specialty of Shoes.

I ALSO DO ELECTROTYPING AT LOWEST RATES.

Address, GEORGE D. RAMSDELL, 65 East Main Street, Rochester, N. Y., U. S. A.

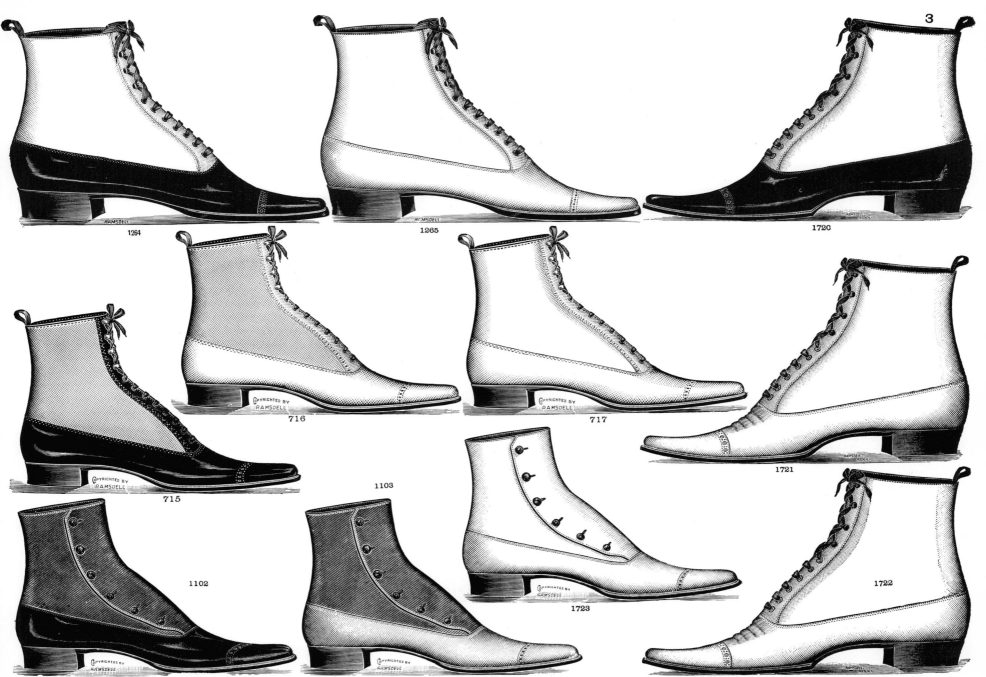

3

1264      1265      1720

715      716      717      1721

1103

1102      1723      1722

**DON'T CUT THEM OUT. ORDER BY NUMBERS.** PRICE $2.00 each for the first one of EACH NUMBER you buy.
EXTRA ELECTROTYPES or DUPLICATES of THAT SAME NUMBER, you can have for 40 cents each.

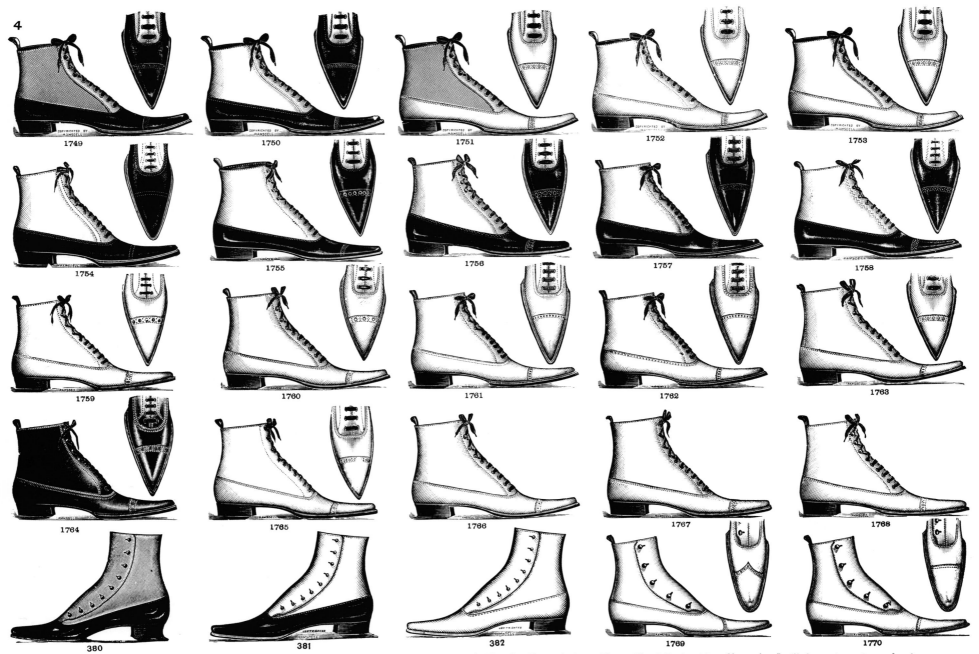

4

1749    1750    1751    1752    1753

1754    1755    1756    1757    1758

1759    1760    1761    1762    1763

1764    1765    1766    1767    1768

380    381    382    1769    1770

These Shoes cost $1.00 each without the front toes.    When the Front toes are left on they cost $1.50 each.    Extra electros with or without the front toes, 20c. each.    I will change toes when ordered.

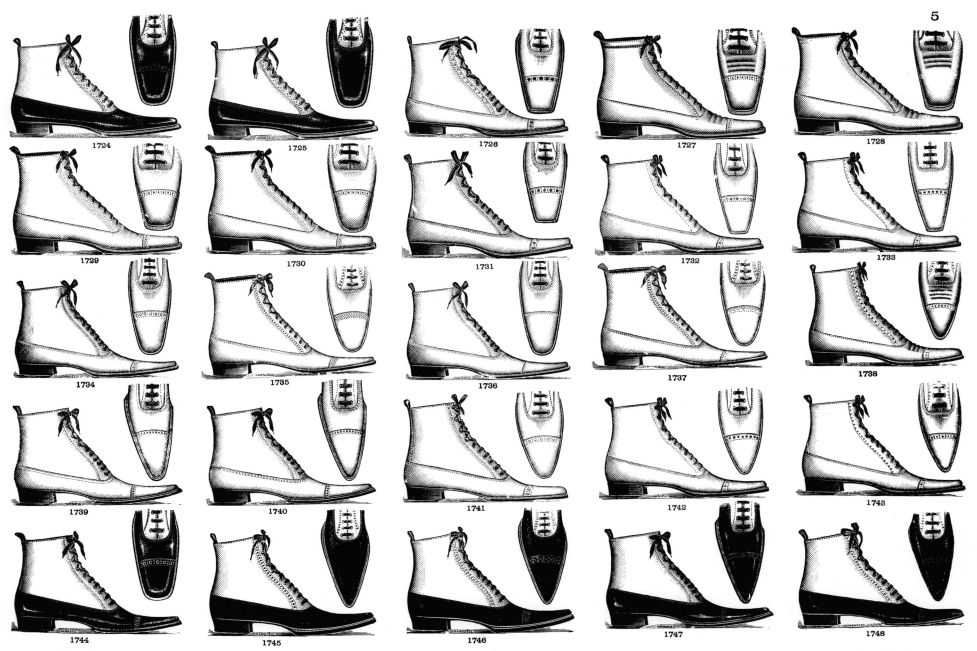

These Shoes cost $1.00 each without the front toes.    When the Front toes are left on they cost $1.50 each.    Extra electros with or without the front toes, 20c. each.    I will change toes when ordered.

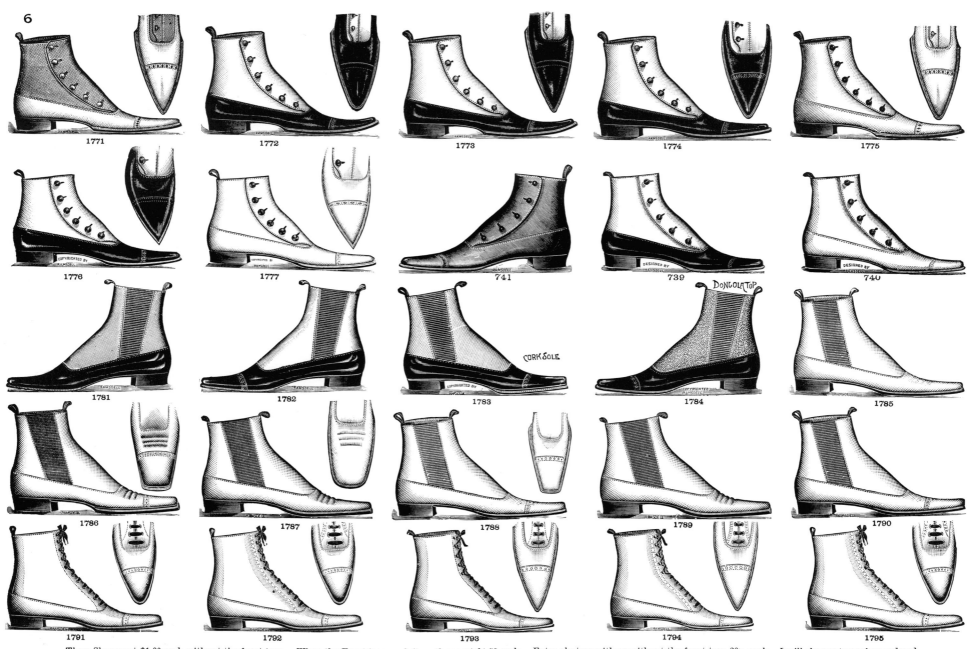

6

1771 1772 1773 1774 1775

1776 1777 741 739 740

1781 1782 1783 1784 1785

1786 1787 1788 1789 1790

1791 1792 1793 1794 1795

These Shoes cost $1.00 each without the front toes.   When the Front toes are left on they cost $1.50 each.   Extra electros with or without the front toes, 20c. each.   I will change toes when ordered.

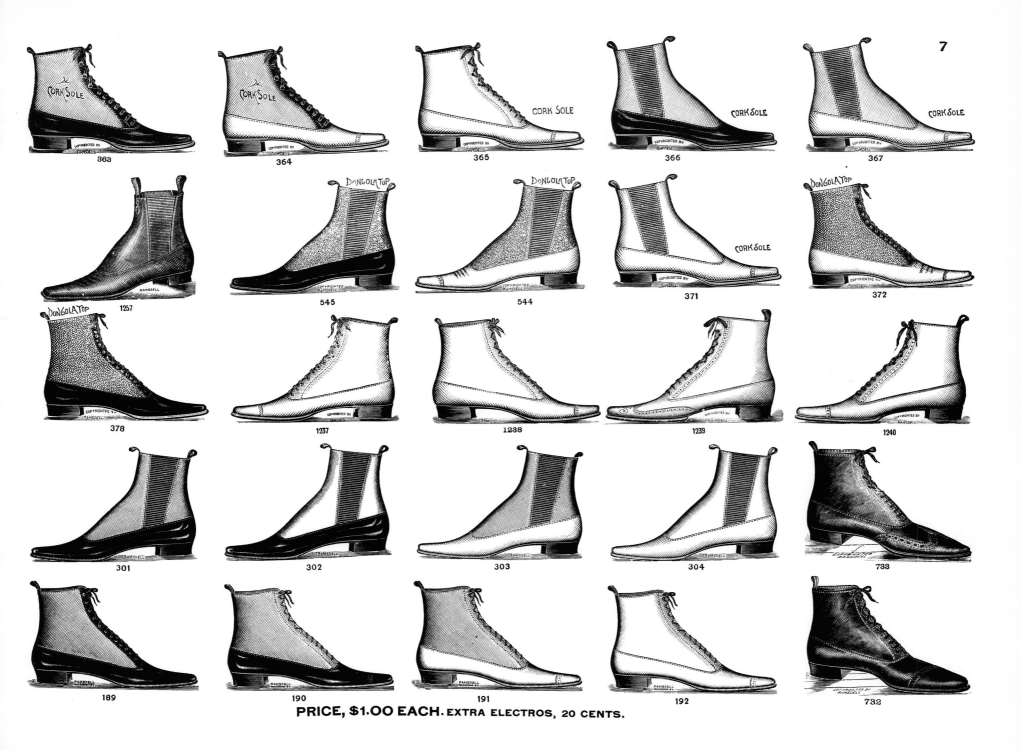

PRICE, $1.00 EACH. EXTRA ELECTROS, 20 CENTS.

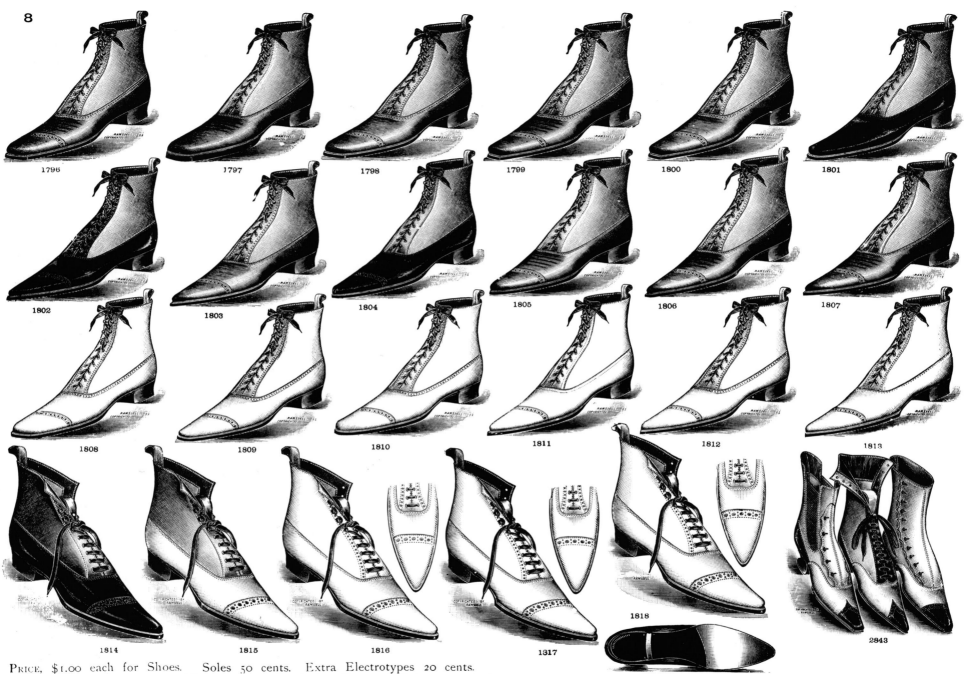

8

1796 1797 1798 1799 1800 1801

1802 1803 1804 1805 1806 1807

1808 1809 1810 1811 1812 1813

1814 1815 1816 1817 1818 2843

PRICE, $1.00 each for Shoes. Soles 50 cents. Extra Electrotypes 20 cents.
When you order Extra Electrotypes and ask for Shoe and Sole on one block, the price for both in this way will be
high Shoes and sole, both on one block. 30 cents. For low Shoes, and soles 25 cents. Remember this applies to extra Electrotypes only.

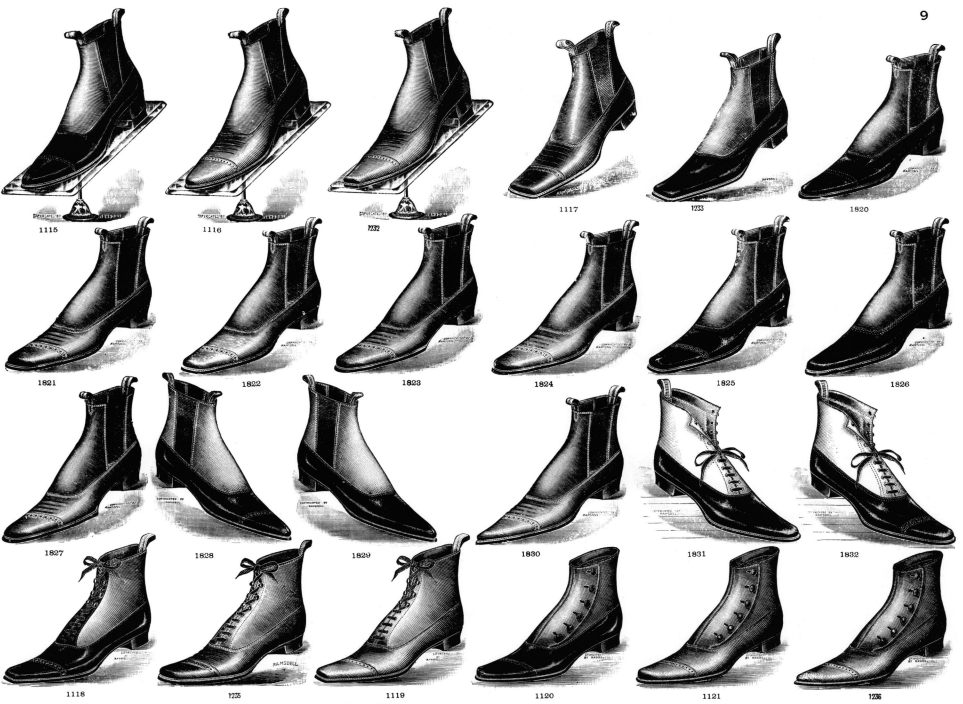

9

1115
1116
1232
1117
1233
1820

1821
1822
1823
1824
1825
1826

1827
1828
1829
1830
1831
1832

1118
1235
1119
1120
1121
1236

PRICE, $1.00 EACH. EXTRA ELECTROS, 20 CENTS.

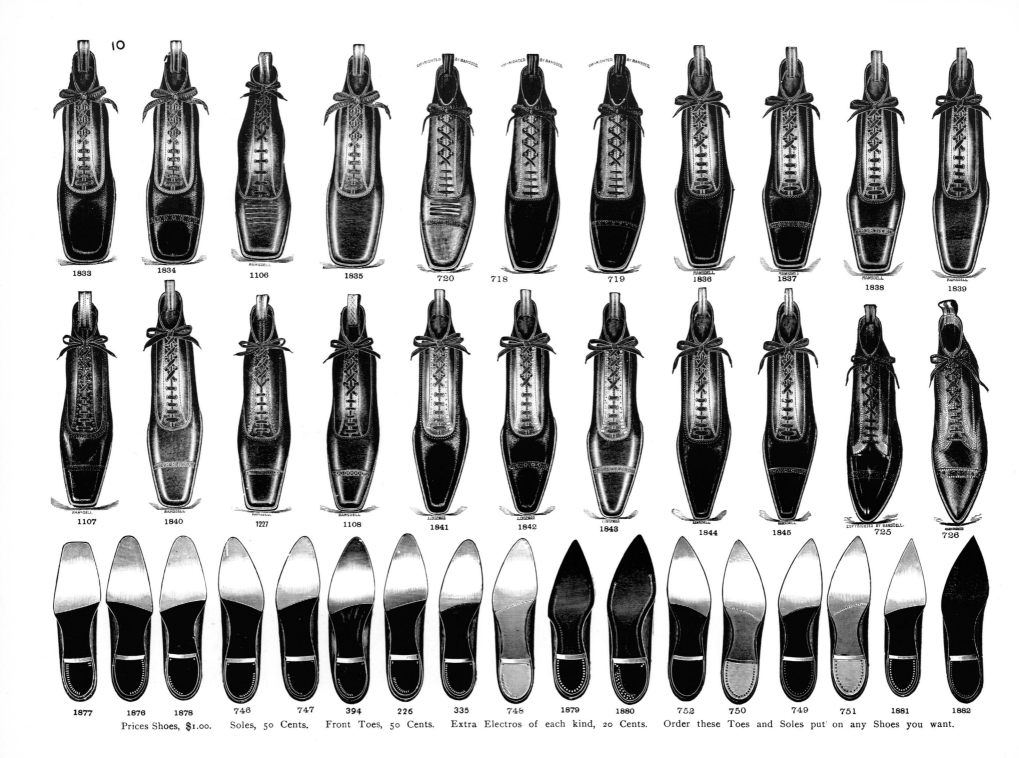

10

1833    1834    1106    1835    720    718    719    1836    1837    1838    1839

1107    1840    1227    1108    1841    1842    1843    1844    1845    725    726

1877    1876    1878    746    747    394    226    335    748    1879    1880    752    750    749    751    1881    1882

Prices Shoes, $1.00.    Soles, 50 Cents.    Front Toes, 50 Cents.    Extra Electros of each kind, 20 Cents.    Order these Toes and Soles put on any Shoes you want.

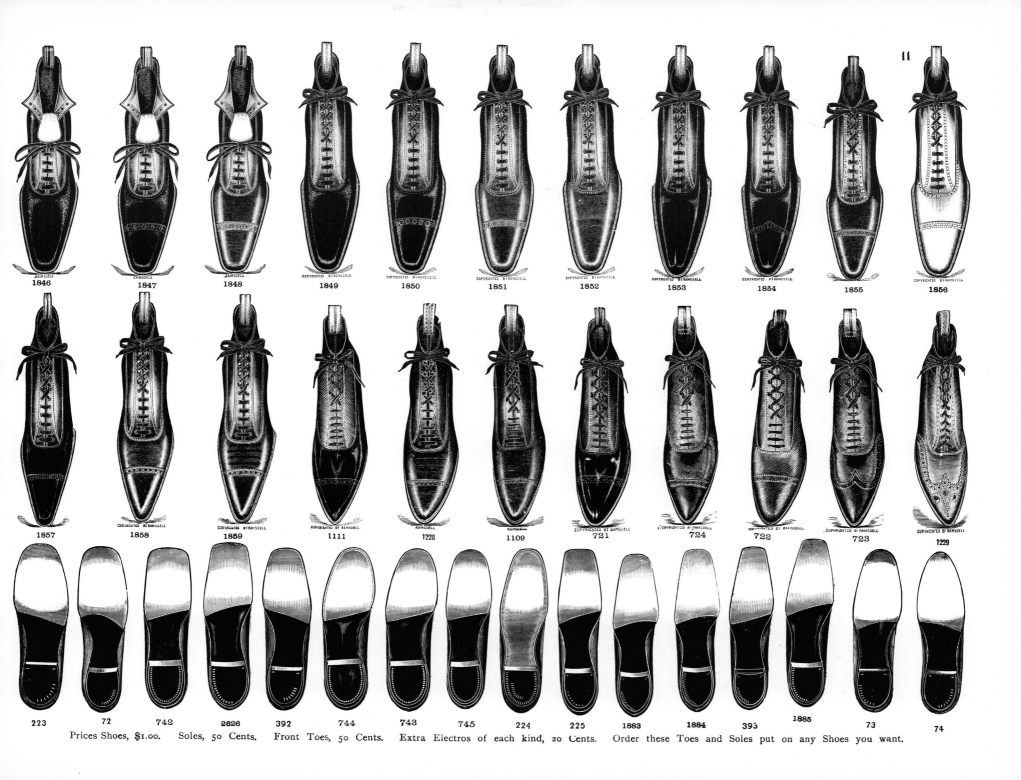

11

1846 1847 1848 1849 1850 1851 1852 1853 1854 1855 1856

1857 1858 1859 1111 1228 1109 721 724 722 723 1229

223 72 742 2626 392 744 743 745 224 225 1883 1884 393 1885 73 74

Prices Shoes, $1.00. Soles, 50 Cents. Front Toes, 50 Cents. Extra Electros of each kind, 20 Cents. Order these Toes and Soles put on any Shoes you want.

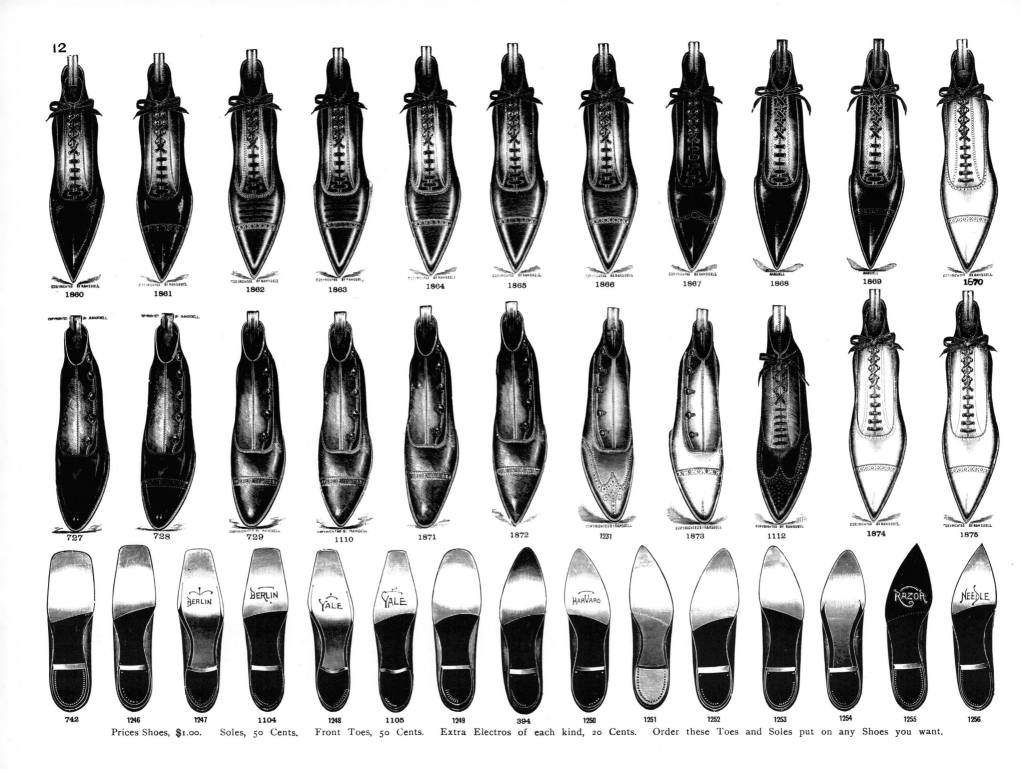

1860 1861 1862 1863 1864 1865 1866 1867 1868 1869 1870

727 728 729 1110 1871 1872 1231 1873 1112 1874 1875

742 1246 BERLIN 1247 BERLIN 1104 YALE 1248 YALE 1105 1249 394 HARVARD 1250 1251 1252 1253 1254 RAZOR 1255 NEEDLE 1256

Prices Shoes, $1.00.     Soles, 50 Cents.     Front Toes, 50 Cents.     Extra Electros of each kind, 20 Cents.     Order these Toes and Soles put on any Shoes you want.

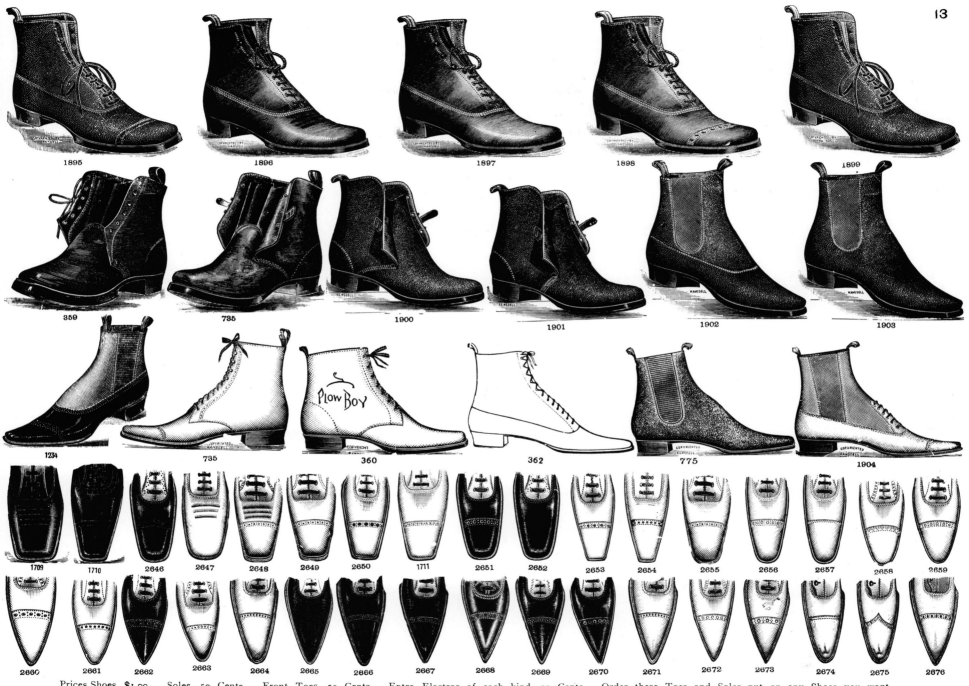

1895    1896    1897    1898    1899

359    735    1900    1901    1902    1903

1234    735    360    362    775    1904

Plow Boy

1709   1710   2646   2647   2648   2649   2650   1711   2651   2652   2653   2654   2655   2656   2657   2658   2659

2660   2661   2662   2663   2664   2665   2666   2667   2668   2669   2670   2671   2672   2673   2674   2675   2676

Prices Shoes, $1.00.    Soles, 50 Cents.    Front Toes, 50 Cents.    Extra Electros of each kind, 20 Cents.    Order these Toes and Soles put on any Shoes you want.

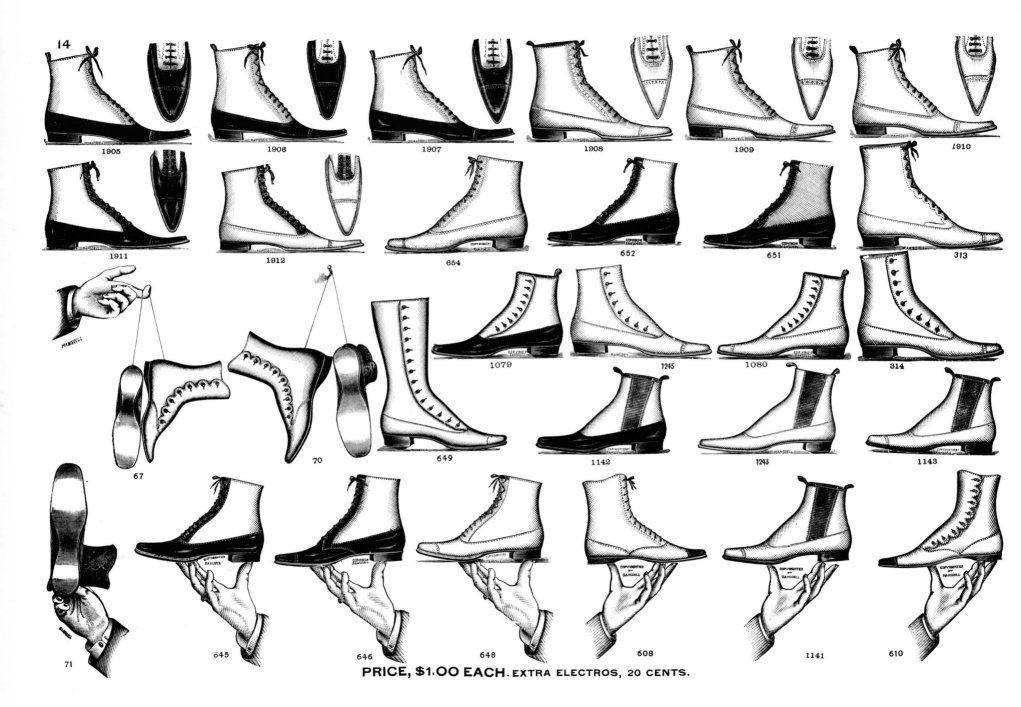

14

1905    1906    1907    1908    1909    1910

1911    1912    654    652    651    313

1079    1245    1080    314

67    70    649    1142    1243    1143

71    645    646    648    608    1141    610

**PRICE, $1.00 EACH. EXTRA ELECTROS, 20 CENTS.**

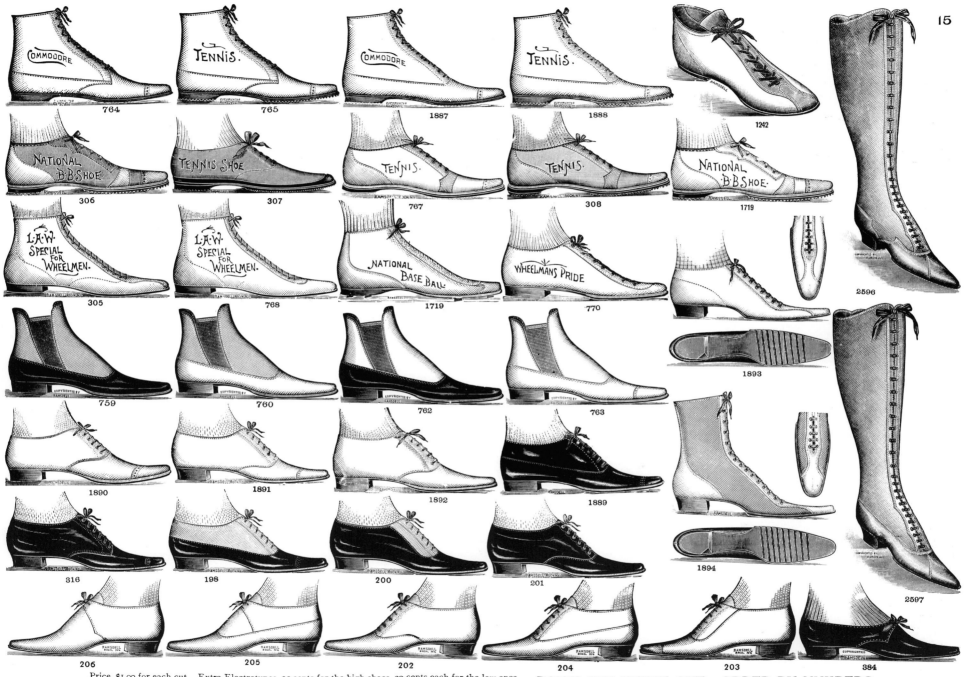

764     765     1887     1888     1242

306     307     767     308     1719

305     768     1719     770     2596

759     760     762     763     1893

1890     1891     1892     1889     1894

316     198     200     201     2597

206     205     202     204     203     384

Price, $1.00 for each cut.    Extra Electrotypes, 20 cents for the high shoes, 20 cents each for the low ones.
Lettering that is on the side of shoe will be taken out if so ordered.    **SOLES, 50 CENTS.**      **DON'T CUT THESE OUT.    ORDER BY NUMBERS.**

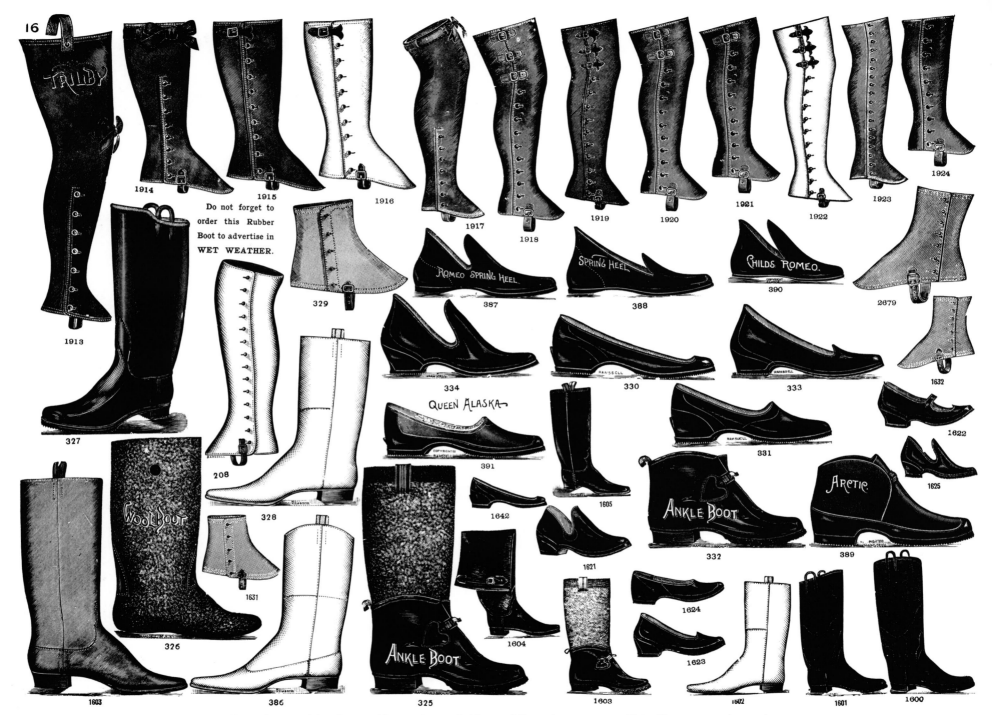

16

TRILBY

Do not forget to
order this Rubber
Boot to advertise in
WET WEATHER.

1914

1915

1916

1917

1918

1919

1920

1921

1922

1923

1924

ROMEO SPRING HEEL

SPRING HEEL

CHILDS ROMEO.

387

388

390

2679

334

330

333

1632

329

1913

327

208

328

326

1631

386

325

QUEEN ALASKA

391

1605

1642

1604

1621

1624

1623

331

1622

1625

ANKLE BOOT

332

ARCTIC.

389

WOOLBOOT

ANKLE BOOT

1603

ANKLE BOOT

1603

1602

1601

1600

All large Boots and Leggings on this page $1.00.    Rubbers and Overgaiters, 50 cents.    Extra Electros, 20 and 25 cents.

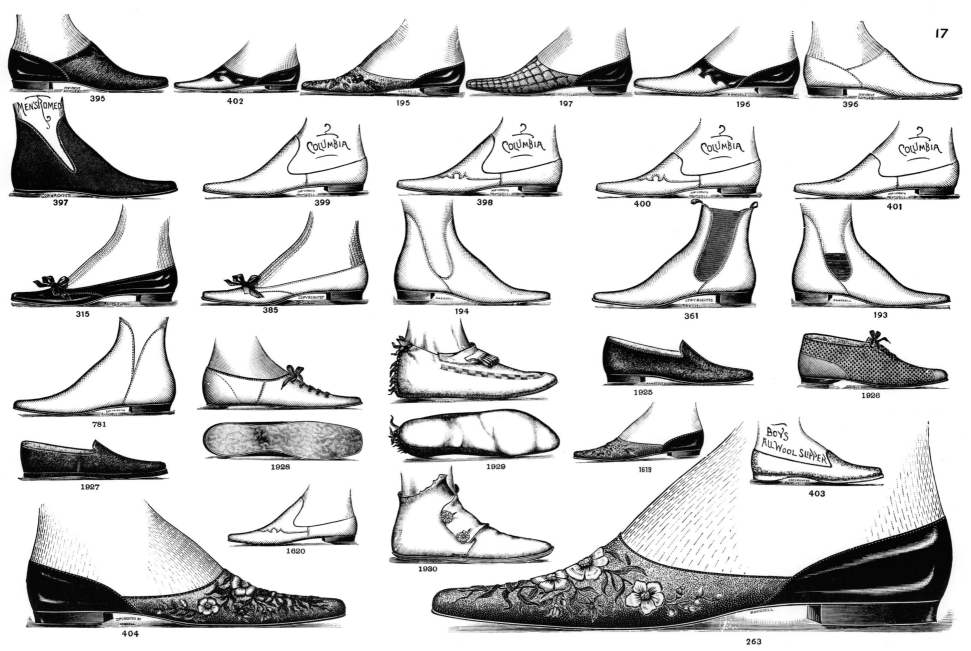

395    402    195    197    196    396

MEN'S ROMEO

397    399    398    400    401

315    385    194    361    193

781    1925    1926

1927    1928    1929    1619    BOY'S ALL WOOL SLIPPER    403

404    1620    1930    263

Price $1.00 each.    Extra electrotypes 20 cents each, except for the two large ones.    Slipper No. 263 which is $2.00 ; extra electros, 65 cents.    No. 404 $1.50 ; extra electros, 35 cents.    (Any body found copying my cuts in this book or my outline designs that are COPYRIGHTED will be prosecuted.)

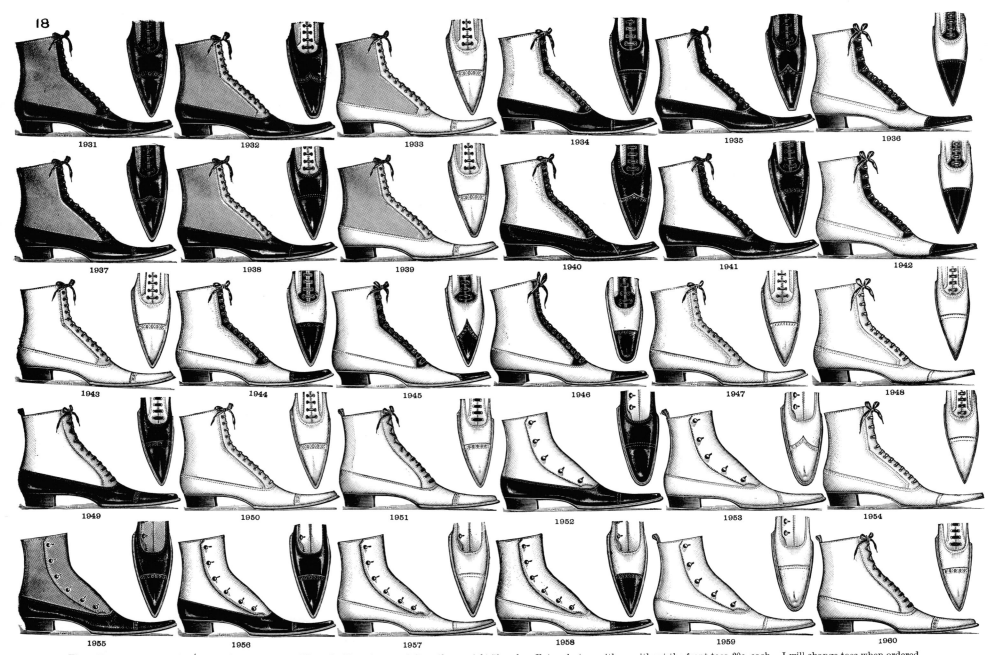

1931 1932 1933 1934 1935 1936
1937 1938 1939 1940 1941 1942
1943 1944 1945 1946 1947 1948
1949 1950 1951 1952 1953 1954
1955 1956 1957 1958 1959 1960

These Shoes cost $1.00 each without the front toes.    When the Front toes are left on they cost $1.50 each.    Extra electros with or without the front toes, 20c. each.    I will change toes when ordered.

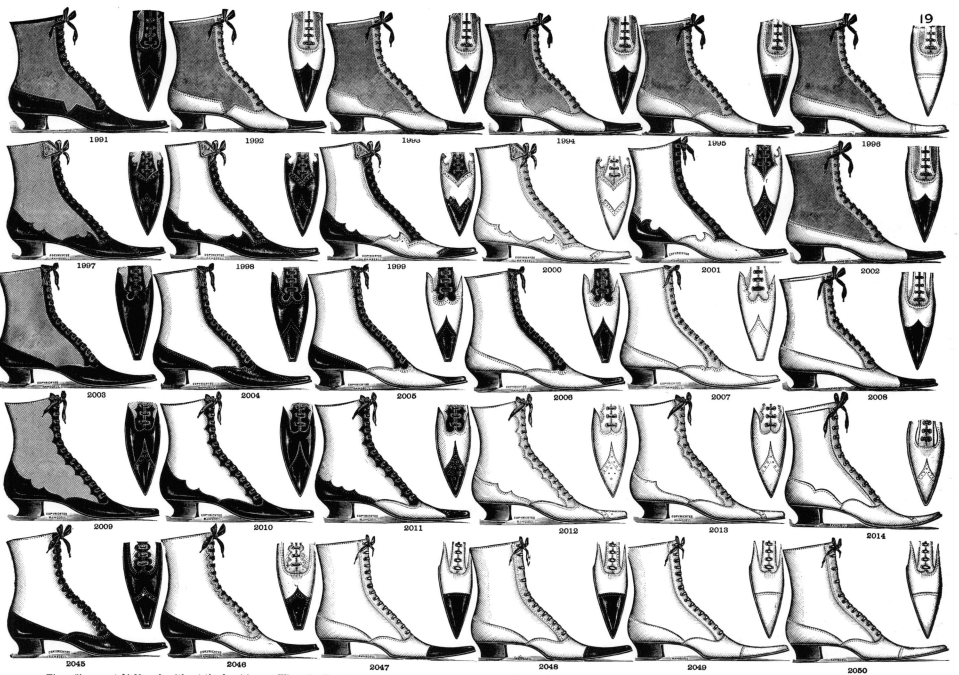

These Shoes cost $1.00 each without the front toes.   When the Front toes are left on they cost $1.50 each.   Extra electros with or without the front toes, 20c. each.   I will change toes when ordered.

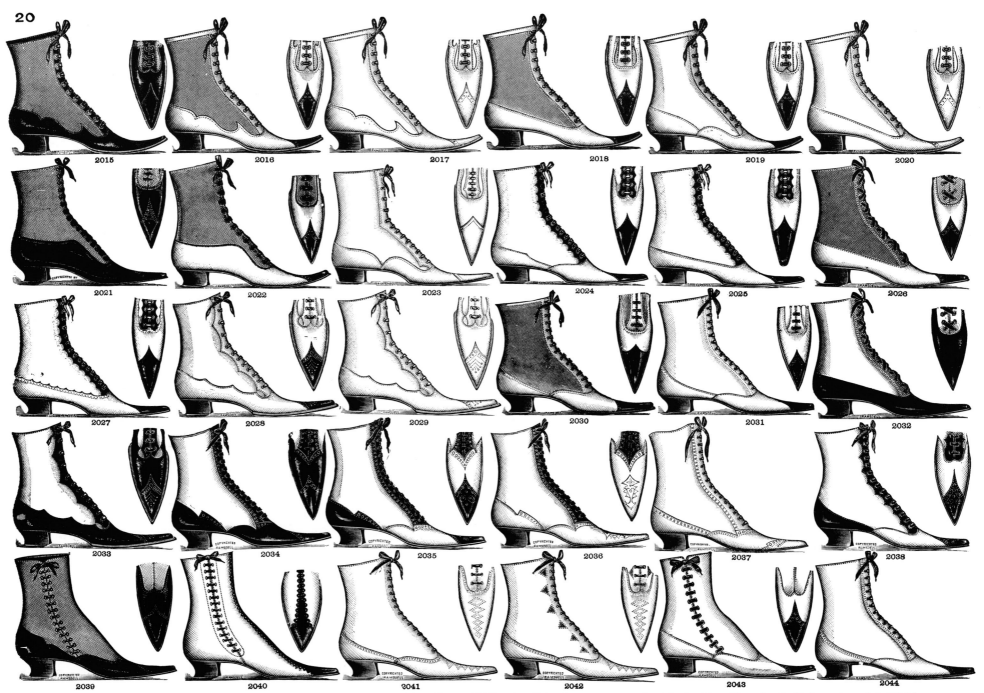

2015   2016   2017   2018   2019   2020
2021   2022   2023   2024   2025   2026
2027   2028   2029   2030   2031   2032
2033   2034   2035   2036   2037   2038
2039   2040   2041   2042   2043   2044

These Shoes cost $1.00 each without the front toes.   When the Front toes are left on they cost $1.50 each.   Extra electros with or without the front toes, 20c. each.   I will change toes when ordered.

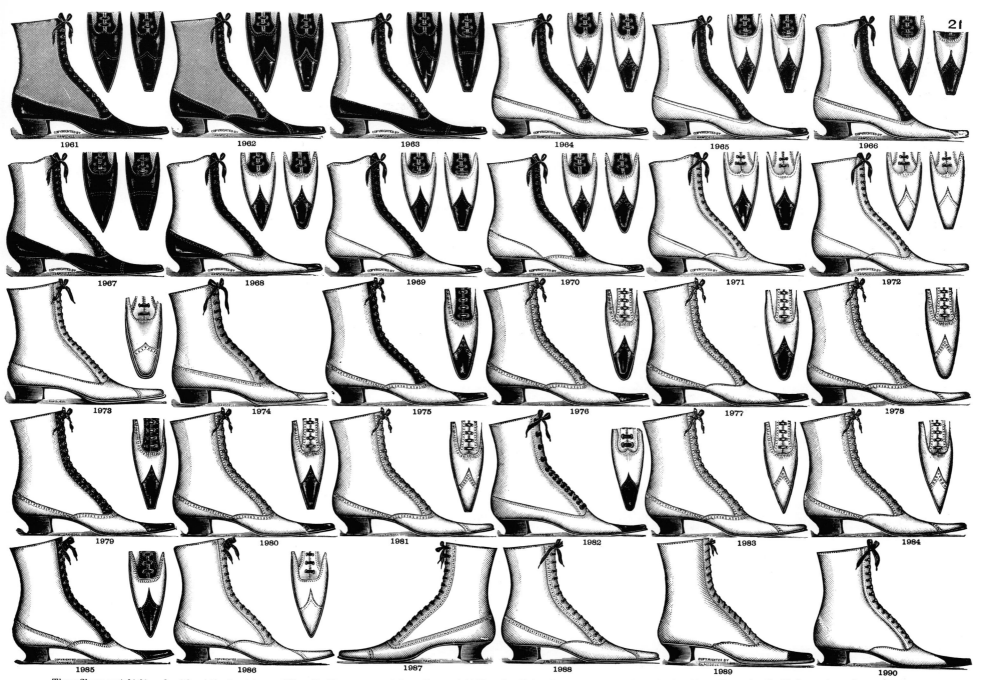

21

1961    1962    1963    1964    1965    1966

1967    1968    1969    1970    1971    1972

1973    1974    1975    1976    1977    1978

1979    1980    1981    1982    1983    1984

1985    1986    1987    1988    1989    1990

These Shoes cost $1.00 each without the front toes.    When the Front toes are left on they cost $1.50 each.    Extra electros with or without the front toes, 20c. each.    I will change toes when ordered.

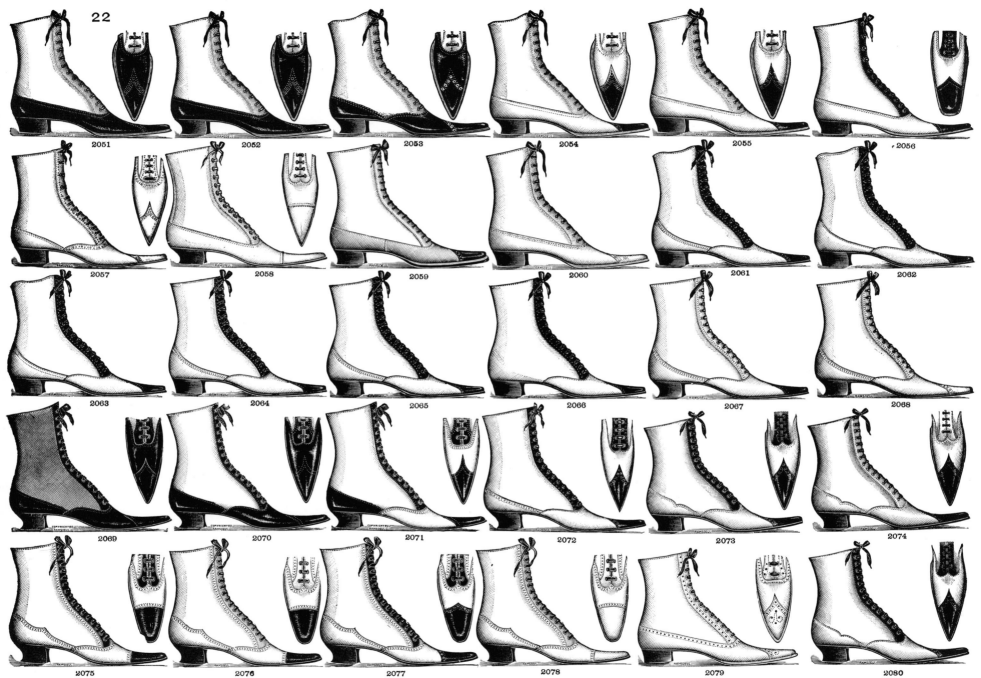

2051    2052    2053    2054    2055    2056

2057    2058    2059    2060    2061    2062

2063    2064    2065    2066    2067    2068

2069    2070    2071    2072    2073    2074

2075    2076    2077    2078    2079    2080

These Shoes cost $1.00 each without the front toes.    When the Front toes are left on they cost $1.50 each.    Extra electros with or without the front toes, 20c. each.    I will change toes when ordered.

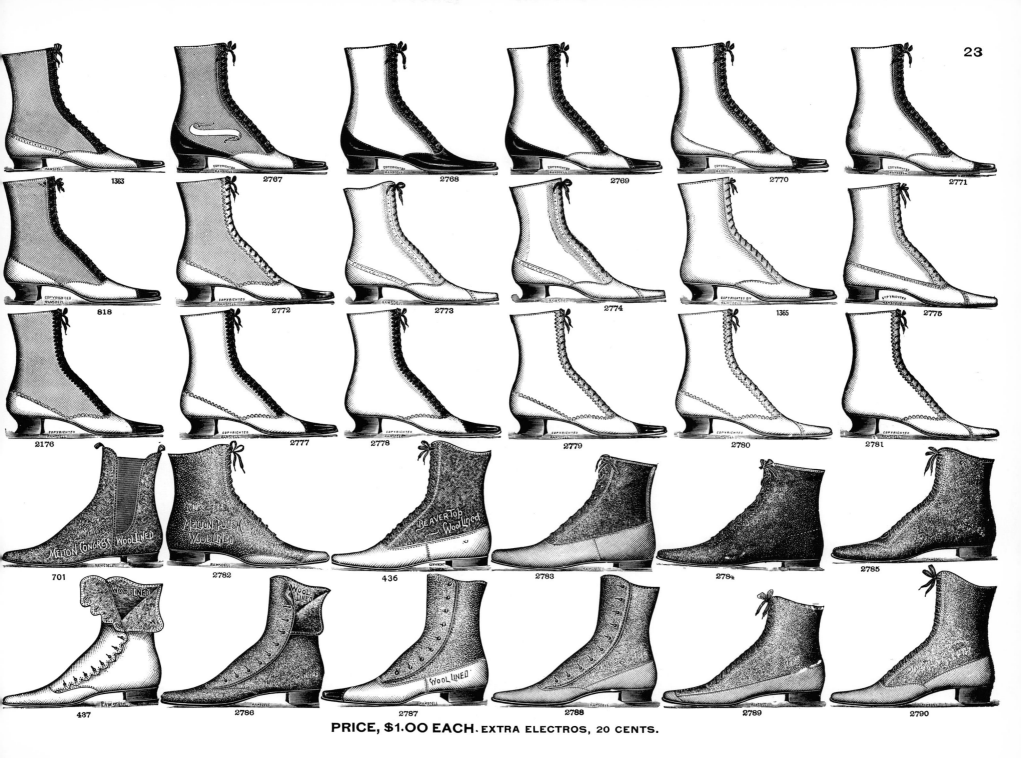

1363    2767    2768    2769    2770    2771

818    2772    2773    2774    1365    2775

2176    2777    2778    2779    2780    2781

701    2782    436    2783    2784    2785

437    2786    2787    2788    2789    2790

**PRICE, $1.00 EACH.** EXTRA ELECTROS, 20 CENTS.

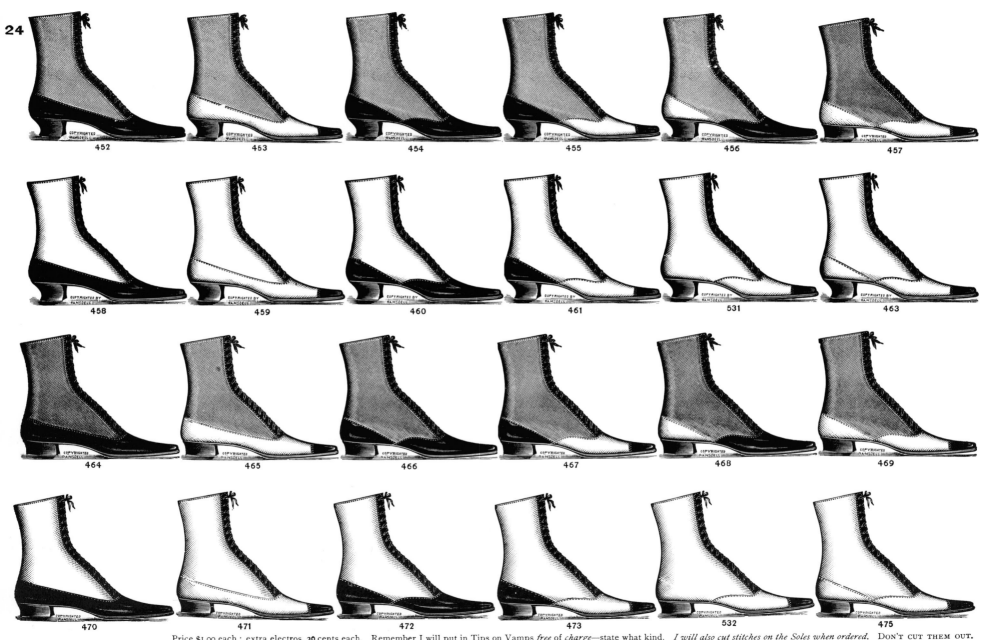

24

452    453    454    455    456    457
458    459    460    461    531    463
464    465    466    467    468    469
470    471    472    473    532    475

Price $1.00 each ; extra electros, **20** cents each.    Remember I will put in Tips on Vamps *free* of *charge*—state what kind.    *I will also cut stitches on the Soles when ordered.*    Don't cut them out.

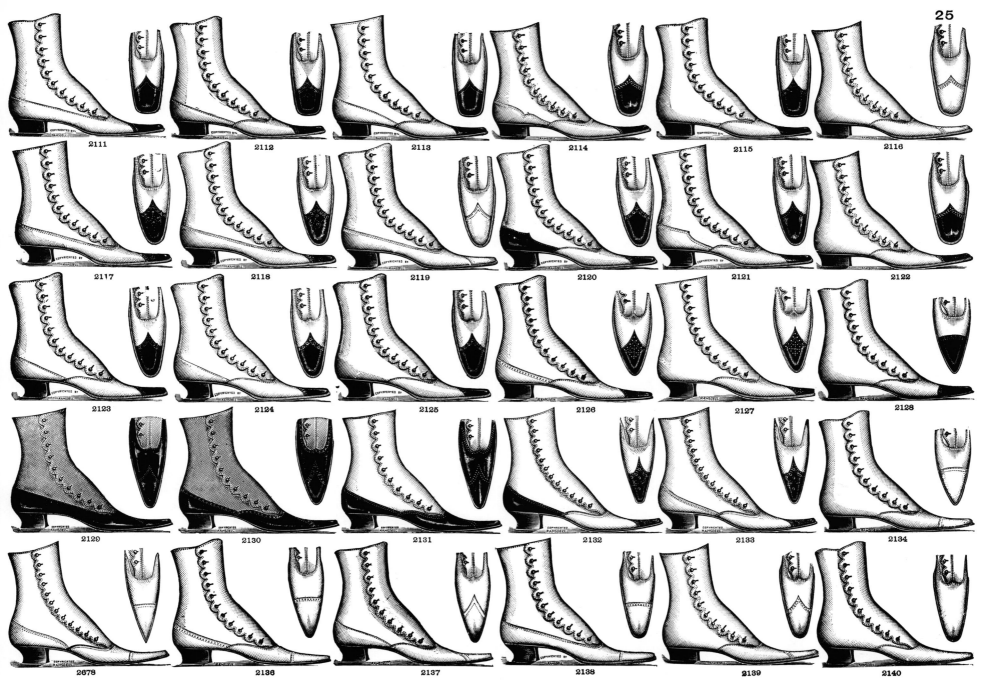

25

2111 2112 2113 2114 2115 2116
2117 2118 2119 2120 2121 2122
2123 2124 2125 2126 2127 2128
2129 2130 2131 2132 2133 2134
2678 2136 2137 2138 2139 2140

These Shoes cost $1.00 each without the front toes.  When the Front toes are left on they cost $1.50 each.  Extra electros with or without the front toes, 20c. each.  I will change toes when ordered.

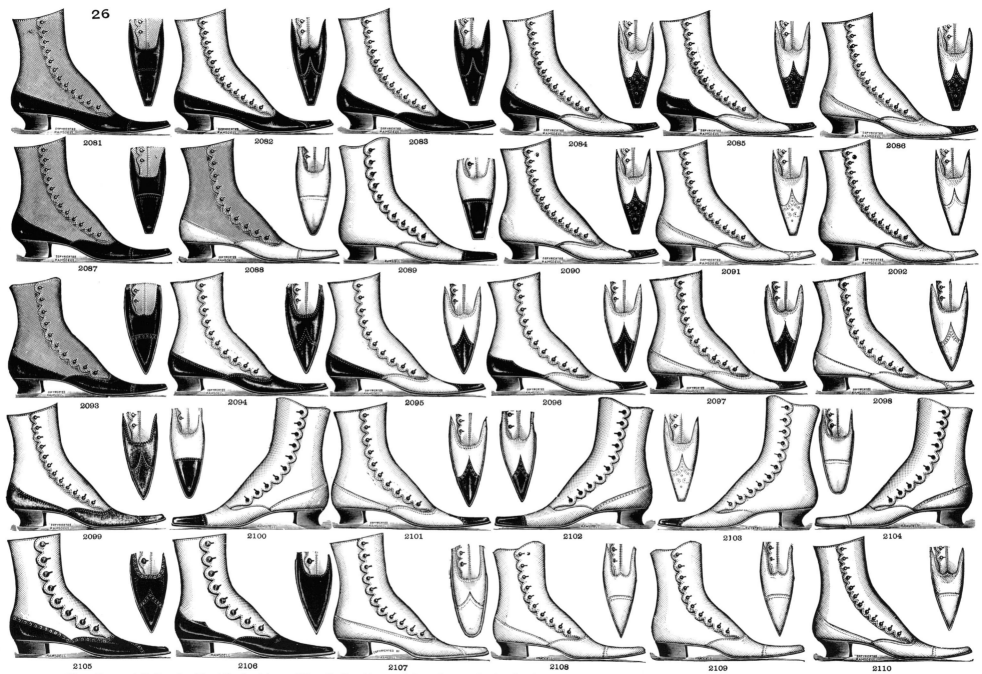

2081    2082    2083    2084    2085    2086

2087    2088    2089    2090    2091    2092

2093    2094    2095    2096    2097    2098

2099    2100    2101    2102    2103    2104

2105    2106    2107    2108    2109    2110

These Shoes cost $1.00 each without the front toes.  When the Front toes are left on they cost $1.50 each.  Extra electros with or without the front toes, 20c. each.  I will change toes when ordered.

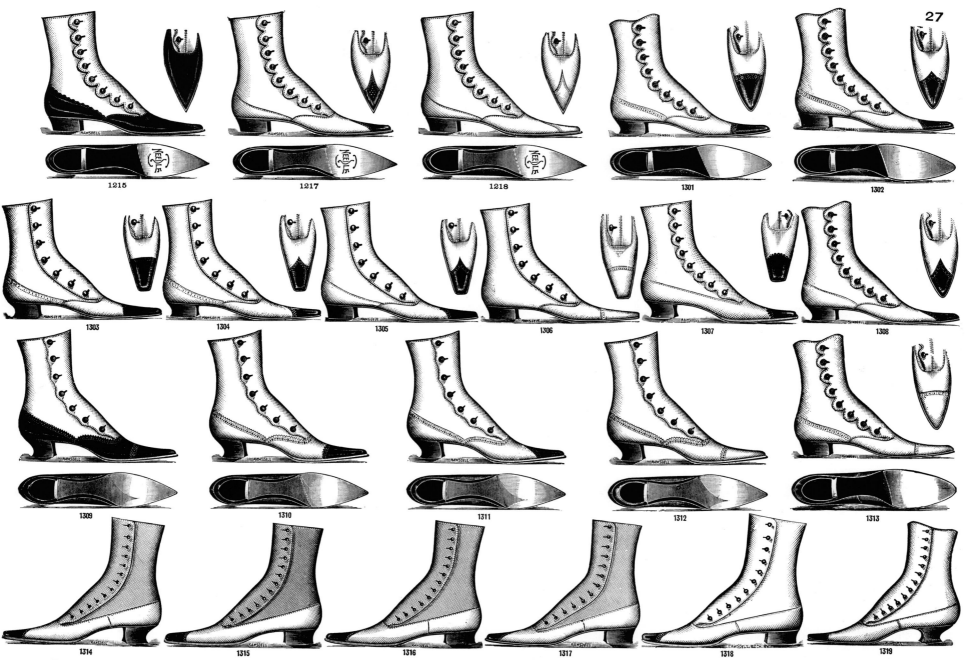

These Shoes cost $1.00 each without the front toes.   When the Front toes are left on they cost $1.50 each.   Extra electros with or without the front toes, 20c. each.   I will change toes when ordered.

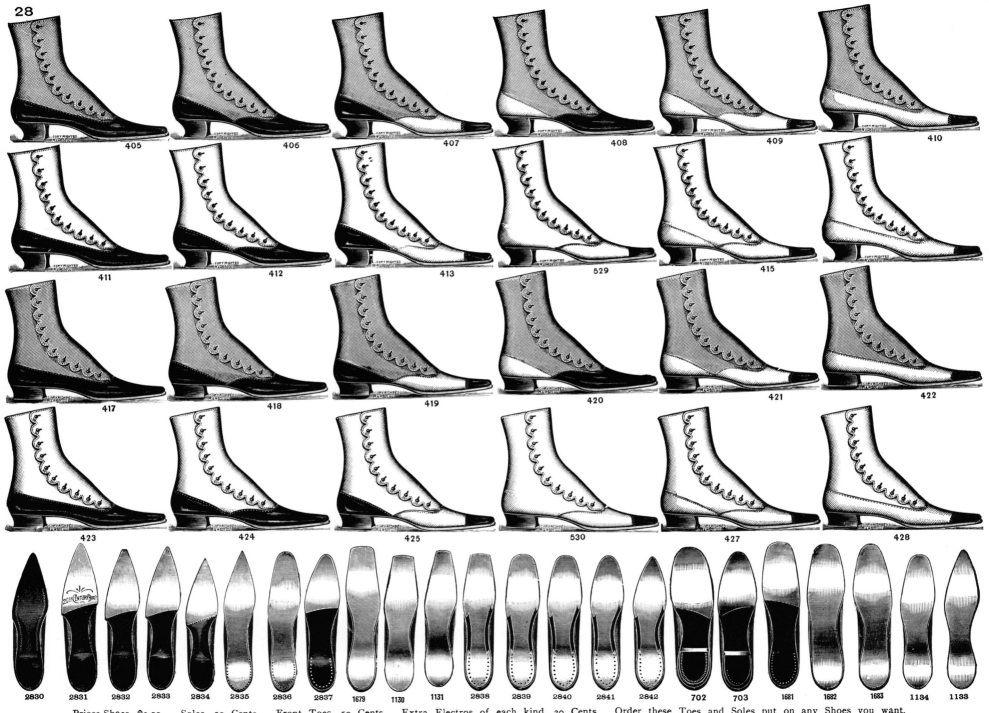

405    406    407    408    409    410

411    412    413    529    415   

417    418    419    420    421    422

423    424    425    530    427    428

2830   2831   2832   2833   2834   2835   2836   2837   1679   1130   1131   2838   2839   2840   2841   2842   702   703   1681   1682   1683   1134   1133

Prices Shoes, $1.00.    Soles, 50 Cents.    Front Toes, 50 Cents.    Extra Electros of each kind, 20 Cents.    Order these Toes and Soles put on any Shoes you want.

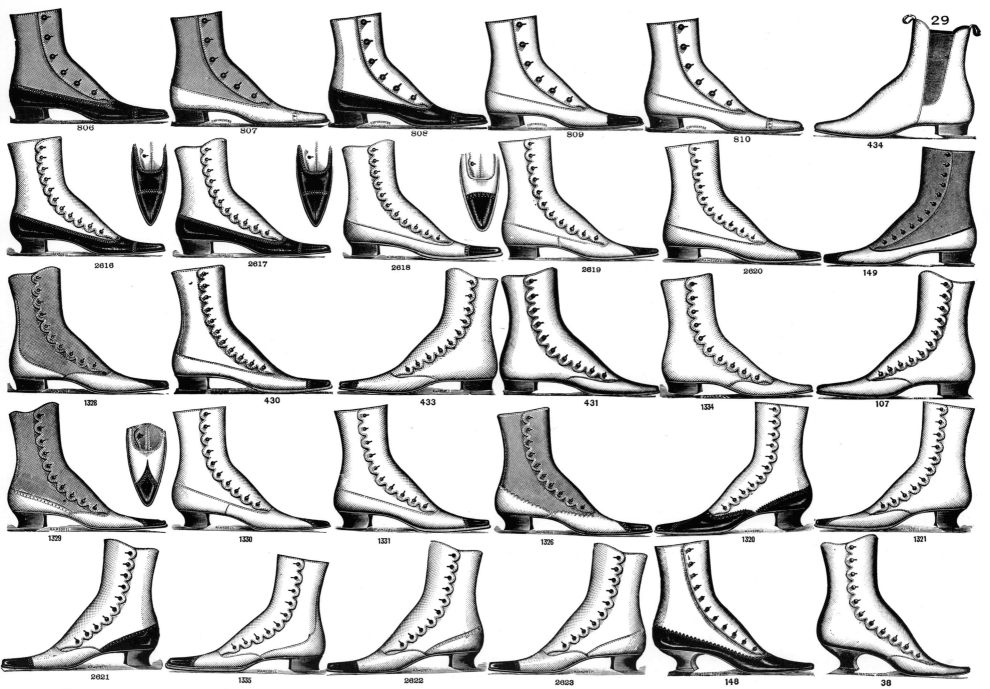

29

806 807 808 809 810 434

2616 2617 2618 2619 2620 149

1328 430 433 431 1334 107

1329 1330 1331 1326 1320 1321

2621 1335 2622 2623 148 38

These Shoes cost $1.00 each without the front toes.    When the Front toes are left on they cost $1.50 each.    Extra electros with or without the front toes, 20c. each.    I will change toes when ordered.

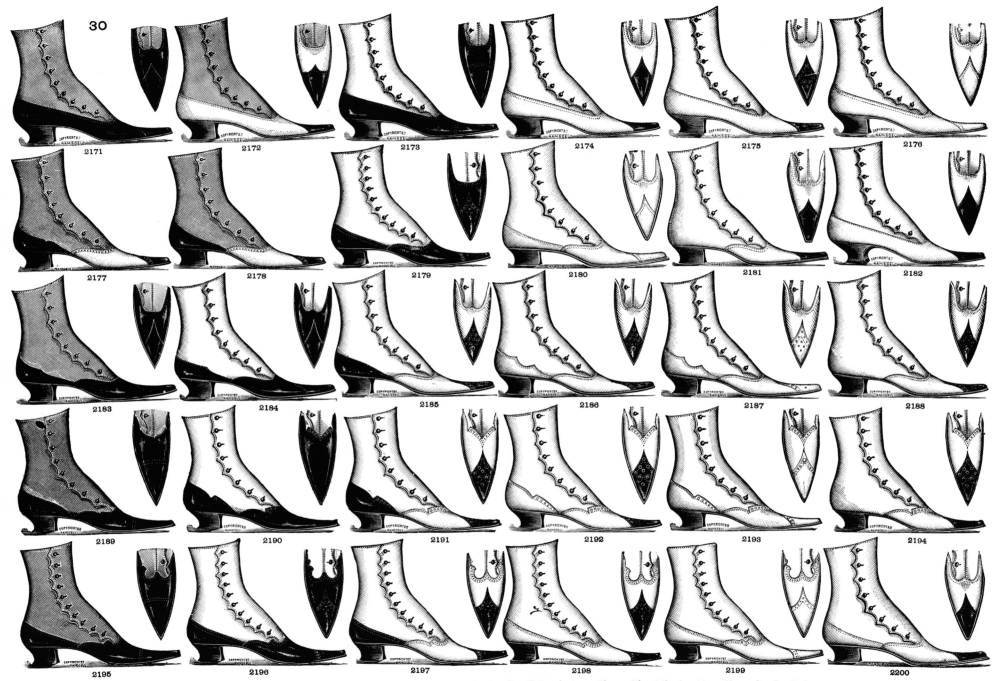

30

2171   2172   2173   2174   2175   2176

2177   2178   2179   2180   2181   2182

2183   2184   2185   2186   2187   2188

2189   2190   2191   2192   2193   2194

2195   2196   2197   2198   2199   2200

These Shoes cost $1.00 each without the front toes.   When the Front toes are left on they cost $1.50 each.   Extra electros with or without the front toes, 20c. each.   I will change toes when ordered.

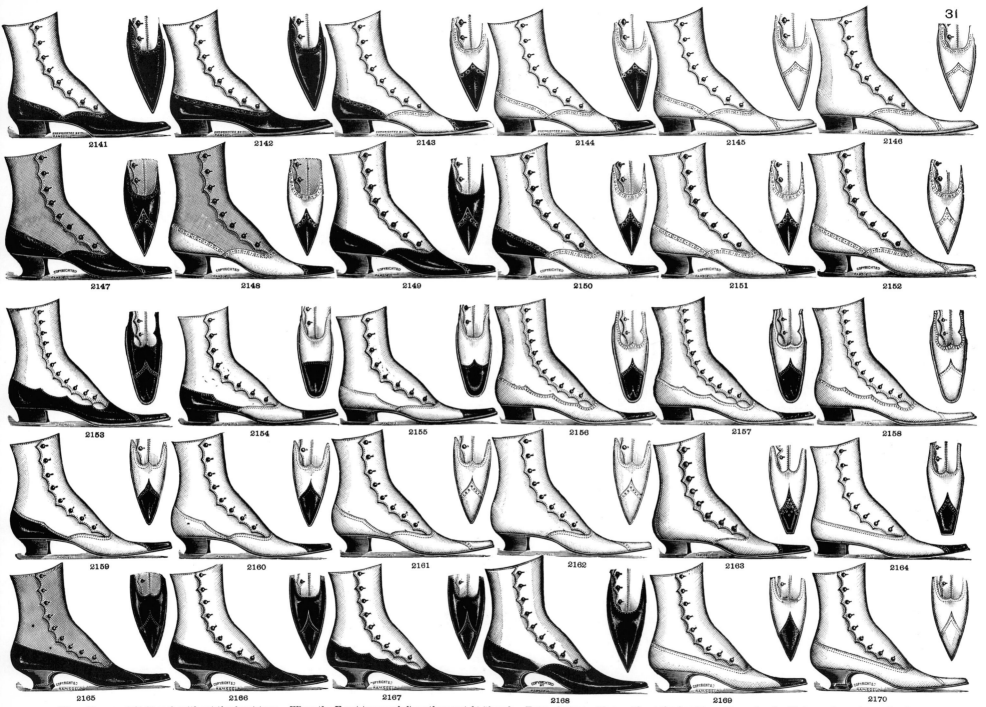

2141   2142   2143   2144   2145   2146

2147   2148   2149   2150   2151   2152

2153   2154   2155   2156   2157   2158

2159   2160   2161   2162   2163   2164

2165   2166   2167   2168   2169   2170

These Shoes cost $1.00 each without the front toes.   When the Front toes are left on they cost $1.50 each.   Extra electros with or without the front toes, 20c. each.   I will change toes when ordered.

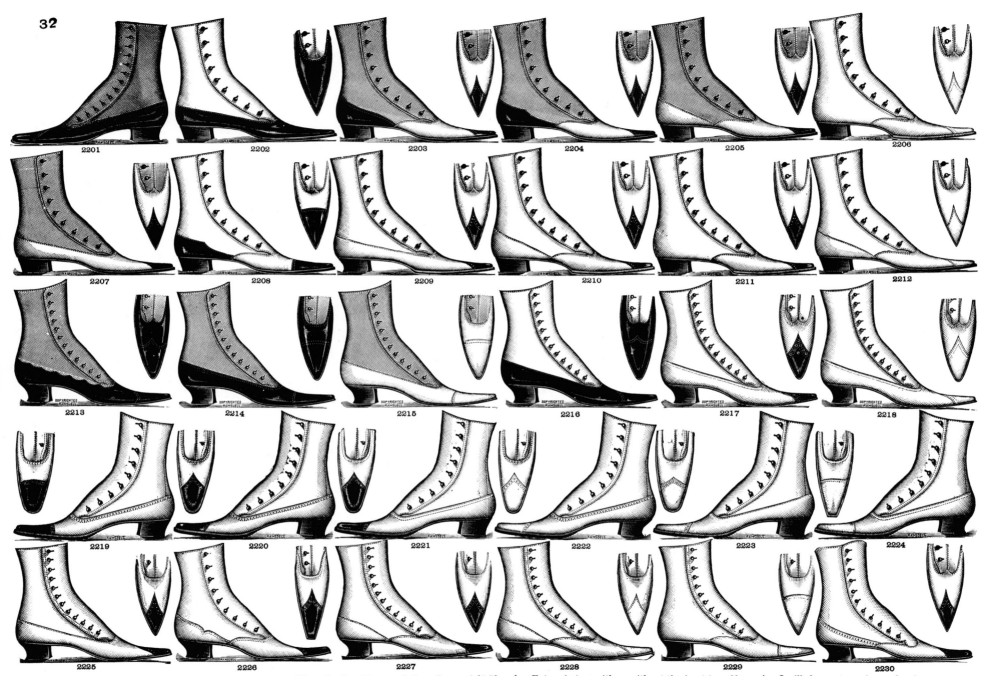

2201 2202 2203 2204 2205 2206
2207 2208 2209 2210 2211 2212
2213 2214 2215 2216 2217 2218
2219 2220 2221 2222 2223 2224
2225 2226 2227 2228 2229 2230

These Shoes cost $1.00 each without the front toes.　　When the Front toes are left on they cost $1.50 each.　　Extra electros with or without the front toes, 20c. each.　　I will change toes when ordered.

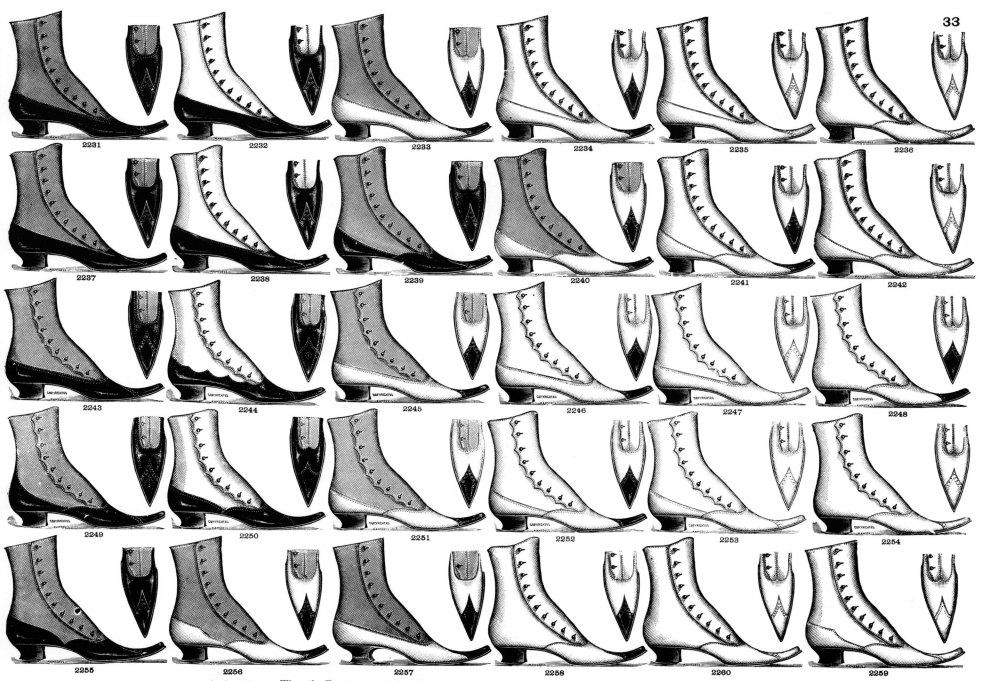

These Shoes cost $1.00 each without the front toes.    When the Front toes are left on they cost $1.50 each.    Extra electros with or without the front toes, 20c. each.    I will change toes when ordered.

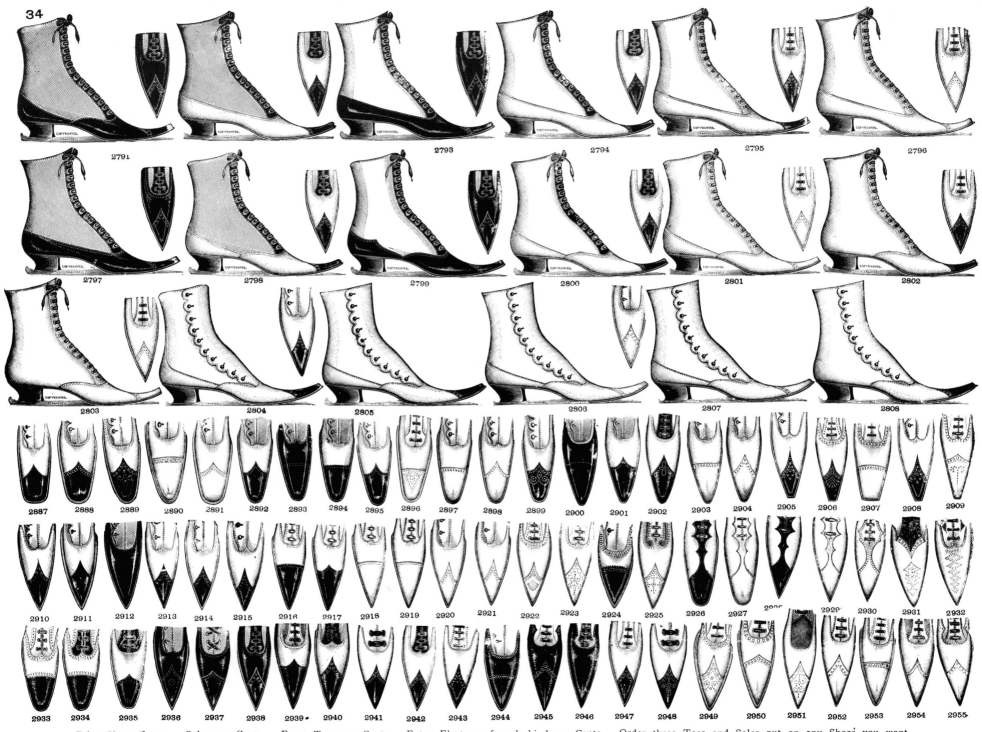

34 Prices Shoes, $1.00. Soles, 50 Cents. Front Toes, 50 Cents. Extra Electros of each kind, 20 Cents. Order these Toes and Soles put on any Shoes you want.

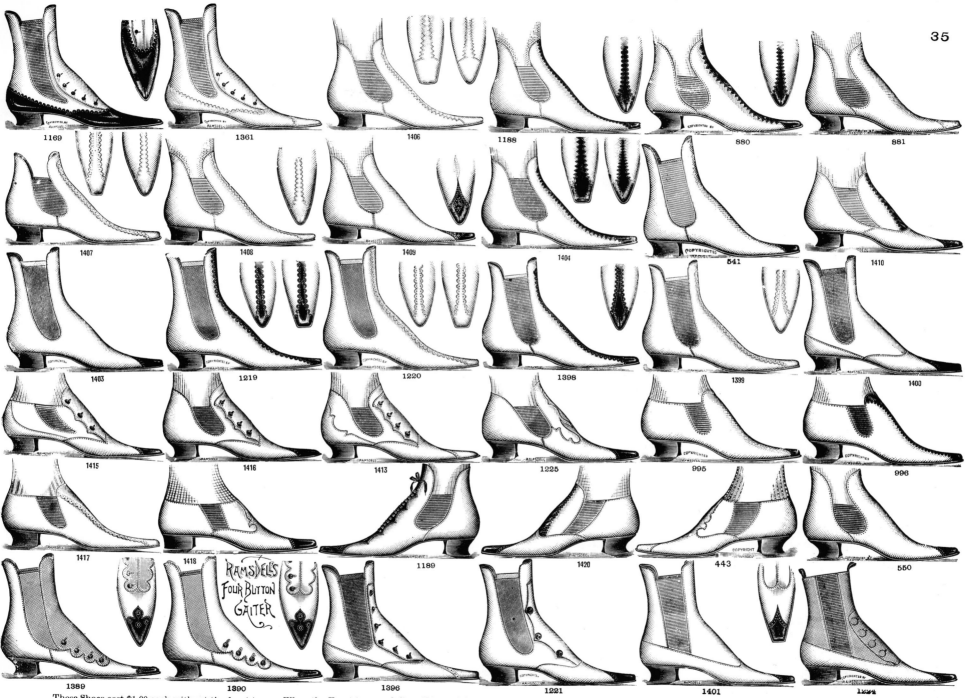

35

1169    1361    1406    1188    880    881

1407    1408    1409    1404    541    1410

1403    1219    1220    1398    1399    1400

1415    1416    1413    1225    995    996

1417    1418    1189    1420    443    550

RAMSDELL'S FOUR BUTTON GAITER

1389    1390    1396    1221    1401    1224

These Shoes cost $1.00 each without the front toes.    When the Front toes are left on they cost $1.50 each.    Extra electros with or without the front toes, 20c. each.    I will change toes when ordered.

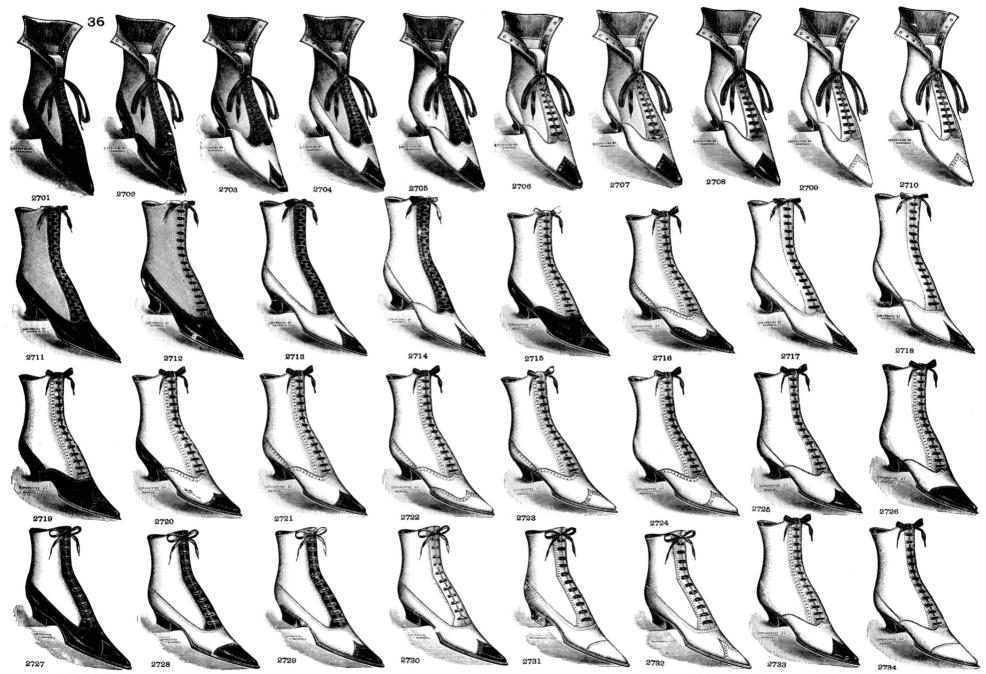

36

2701 2702 2703 2704 2705 2706 2707 2708 2709 2710

2711 2712 2713 2714 2715 2716 2717 2718

2719 2720 2721 2722 2723 2724 2725 2726

2727 2728 2729 2730 2731 2732 2733 2734

**PRICE, $1.OO EACH.** EXTRA ELECTROS, 20 CENTS. (Don't order names on Front View Shoes.) **DON'T CUT THIS BOOK. ORDER BY NUMBERS.**

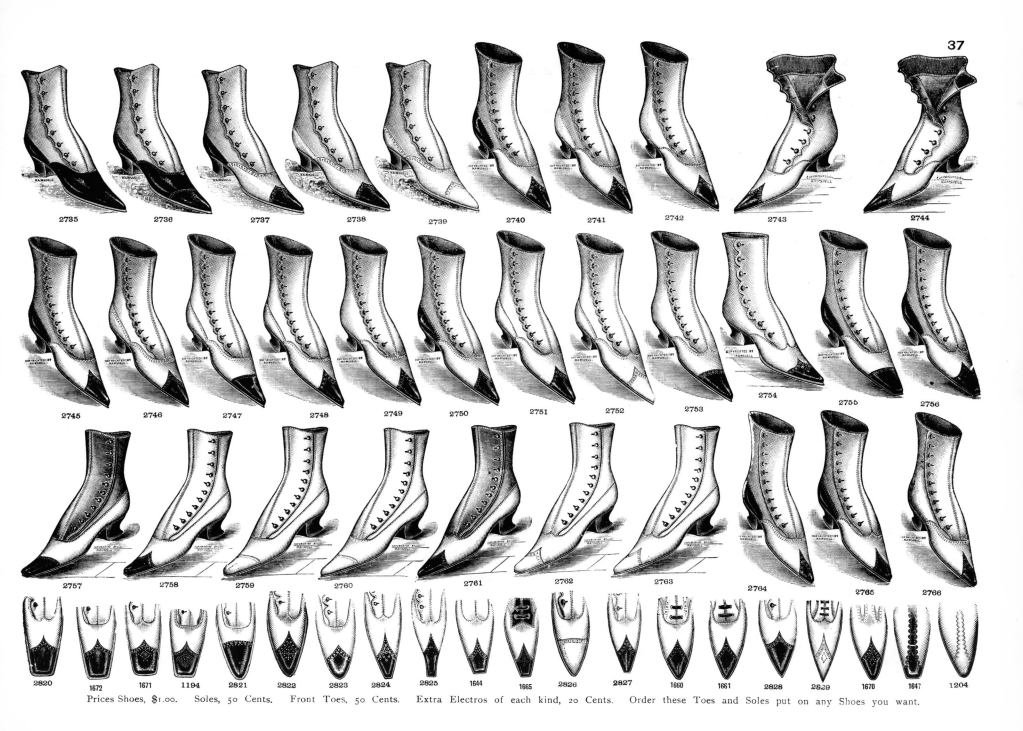

2735    2736    2737    2738    2739    2740    2741    2742    2743    2744

2745    2746    2747    2748    2749    2750    2751    2752    2753    2754    2755    2756

2757    2758    2759    2760    2761    2762    2763    2764    2765    2766

2820   1672   1671   1194   2821   2822   2823   2824   2825   1644   1665   2826   2827   1660   1661   2828   2829   1670   1647   1204

Prices Shoes, $1.00.    Soles, 50 Cents.    Front Toes, 50 Cents.    Extra Electros of each kind, 20 Cents.    Order these Toes and Soles put on any Shoes you want.

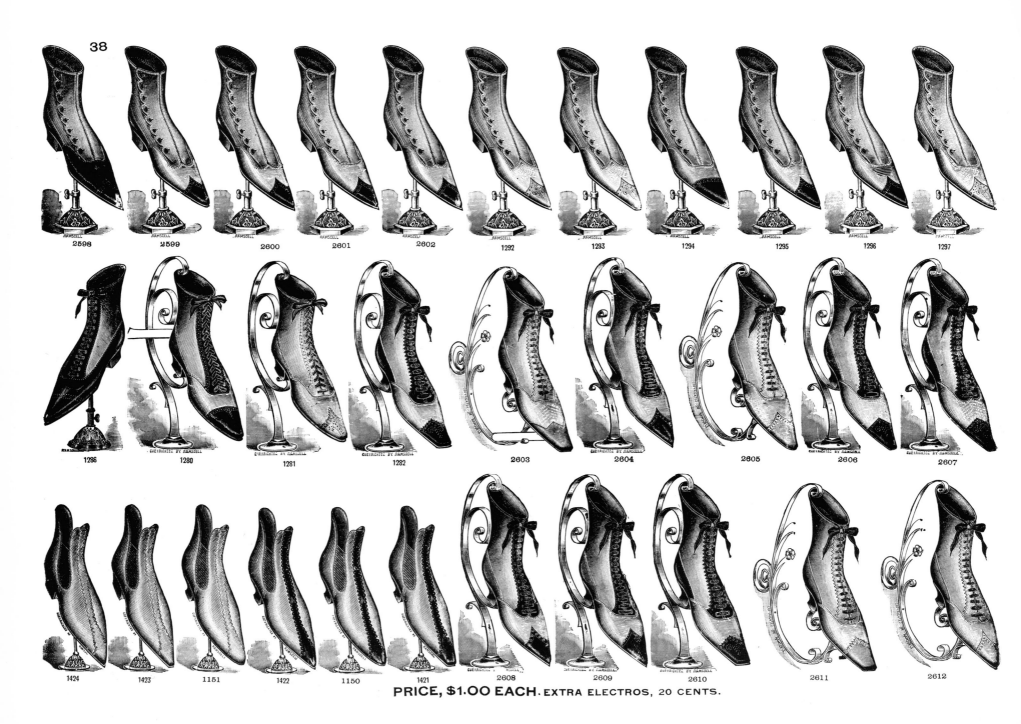

38

2598    2599    2600    2601    2602    1292    1293    1294    1295    1296    1297

1286    1280    1281    1282    2603    2604    2605    2606    2607

1424    1423    1151    1422    1150    1421    2608    2609    2610    2611    2612

**PRICE, $1.00 EACH.** EXTRA ELECTROS, 20 CENTS.

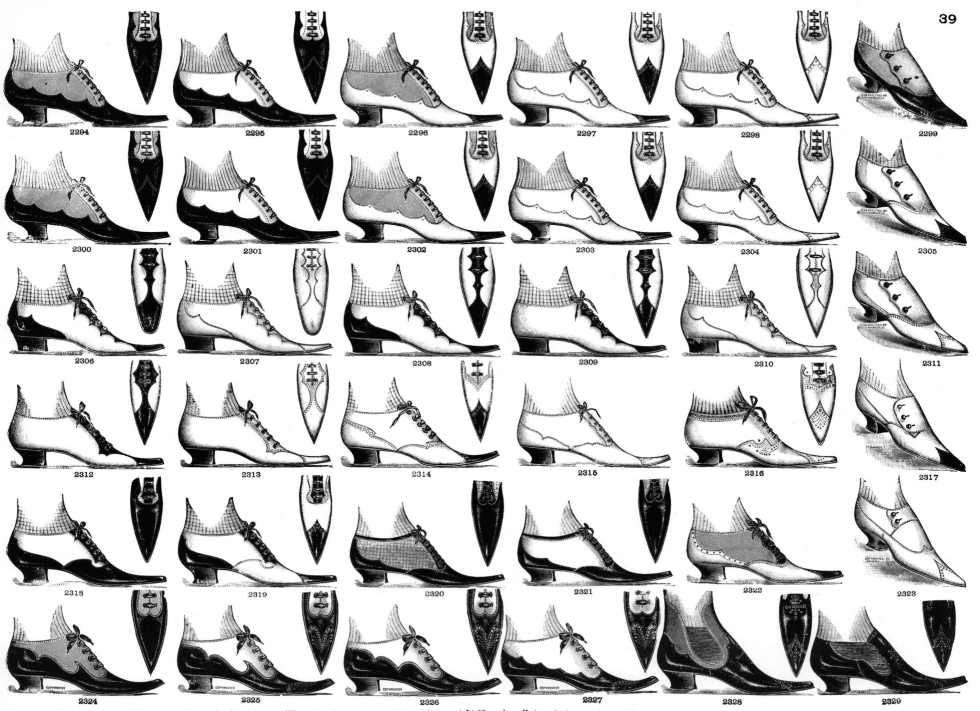

2294    2295    2296    2297    2298    2299

2300    2301    2302    2303    2304    2305

2306    2307    2308    2309    2310    2311

2312    2313    2314    2315    2316    2317

2318    2319    2320    2321    2322    2323

2324    2325    2326    2327    2328    2329

These Shoes cost $1.00 each without the front toes.    When the Front toes are left on they cost $1.50 each.    Extra electros with or without the front toes, 20c. each.    I will change toes when ordered.

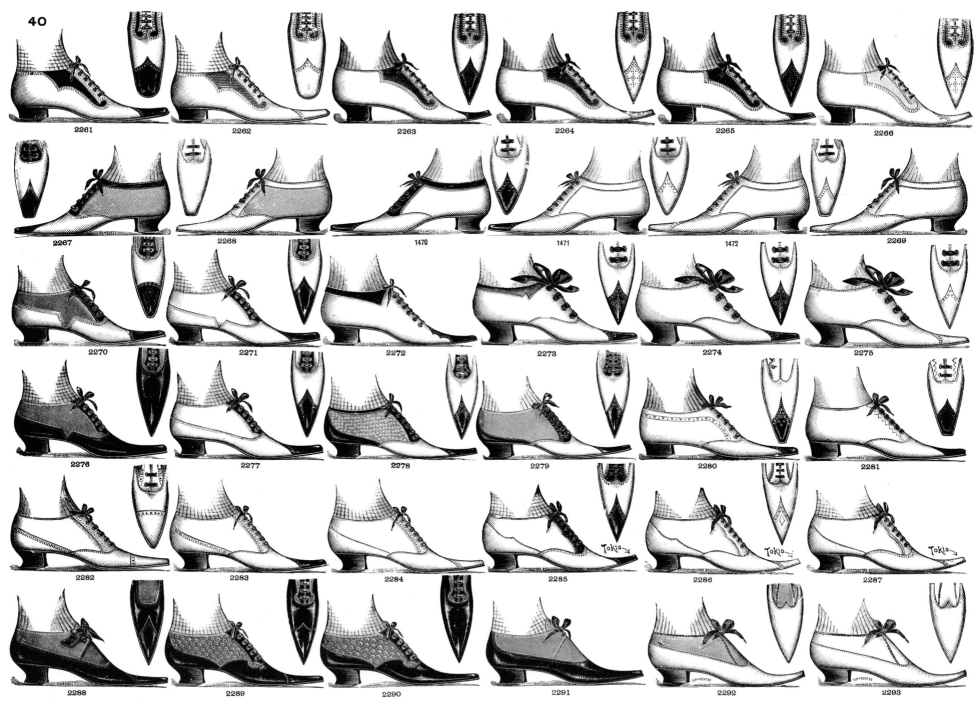

40

2261 2262 2263 2264 2265 2266

2267 2268 1470 1471 1472 2269

2270 2271 2272 2273 2274 2275

2276 2277 2278 2279 2280 2281

2282 2283 2284 2285 2286 2287

2288 2289 2290 2291 2292 2293

These Shoes cost $1.00 each without the front toes.　When the Front toes are left on they cost $1.50 each.　Extra electros with or without the front toes, 20c. each.　I will change toes when ordered.

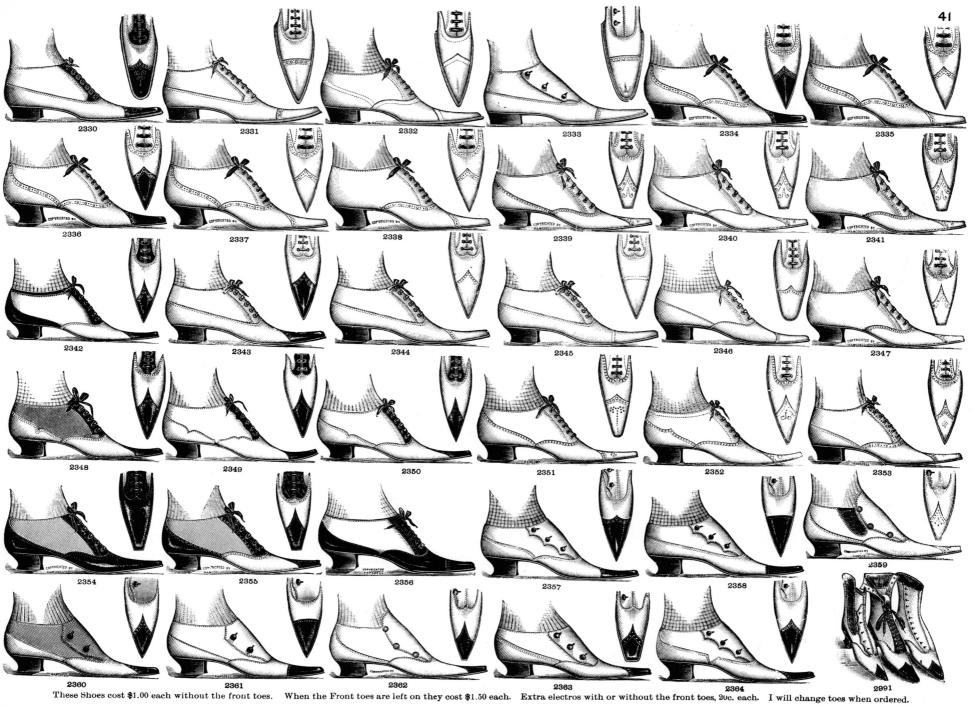

41

These Shoes cost $1.00 each without the front toes.　When the Front toes are left on they cost $1.50 each.　Extra electros with or without the front toes, 20c. each.　I will change toes when ordered.

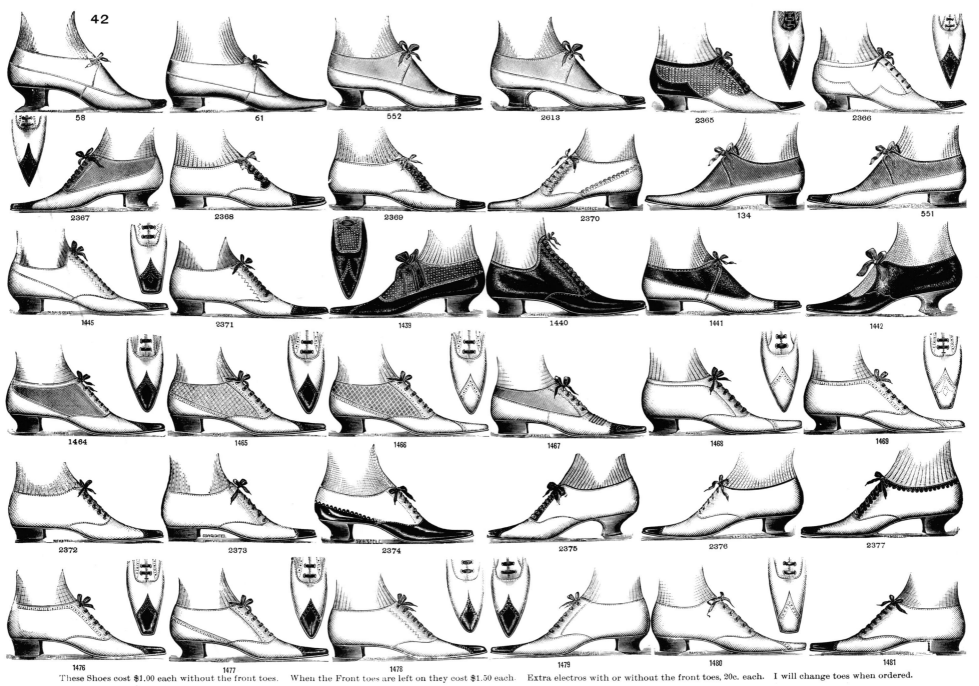

42

58     61     552     2613     2365     2366

2367     2368     2369     2370     134     551

1445     2371     1439     1440     1441     1442

1464     1465     1466     1467     1468     1469

2372     2373     2374     2375     2376     2377

1476     1477     1478     1479     1480     1481

These Shoes cost $1.00 each without the front toes.    When the Front toes are left on they cost $1.50 each.    Extra electros with or without the front toes, 20c. each.    I will change toes when ordered.

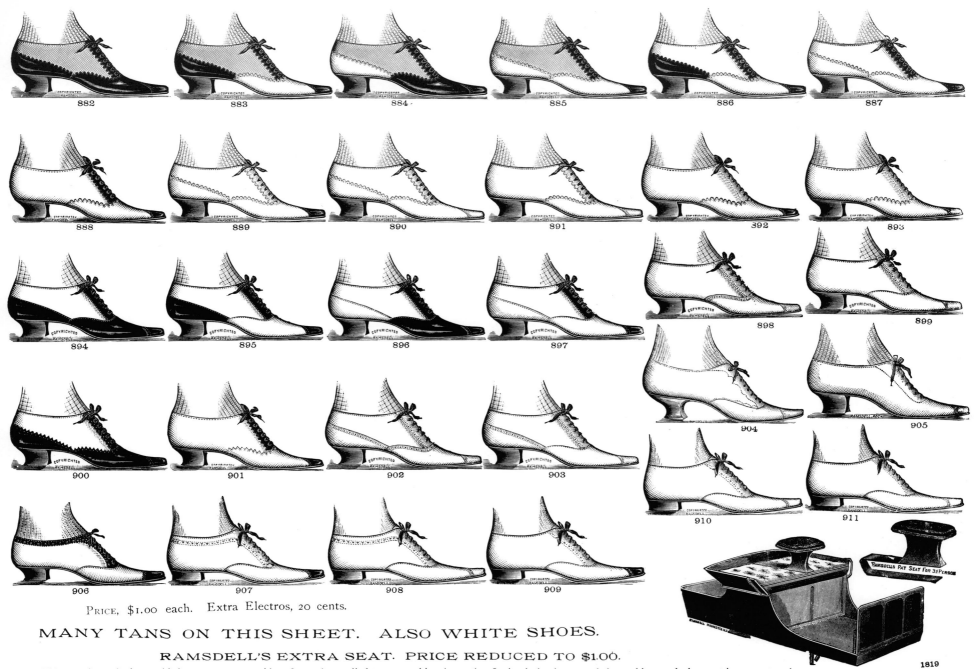

882 883 884 885 886 887

888 889 890 891 392 893

894 895 896 897 898 899

900 901 902 903 904 905

906 907 908 909 910 911

PRICE, $1.00 each.   Extra Electros, 20 cents.

# MANY TANS ON THIS SHEET.   ALSO WHITE SHOES.

## RAMSDELL'S EXTRA SEAT.   PRICE REDUCED TO $1.00.

This seat is used when a third person wants to ride.   It can be applied to any cushion (*see cut*).   It simply hooks around the cushion, and when not in use put under the seat.   Two seconds is time enough to adjust it.   It is the only seat ever invented that can be changed from one vehicle to another without extra fixtures.   All the space that is taken up by this seat is 1¼ inch.   Anybody ordering shoes and this seat can have both shipped under one express charge, with only 10 cents difference in charges.

1819

912 913 914 915 916 917

918 919 920 921 922 923

924 925 926 927 928 929

2397 2398 2399 2400 2401 2402

936 937 938 939 940 941

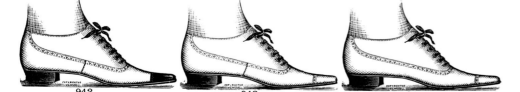

942 943 944

PRICE, $1.00 EACH.

EXTRA ELECTROS, 20 CENTS.

MANY TANS AND WHITE SHOES ON THIS SHEET.

I CAN TAKE OUT PIECE FOXES OR TIPS.

NO EXTRA CHARGE.

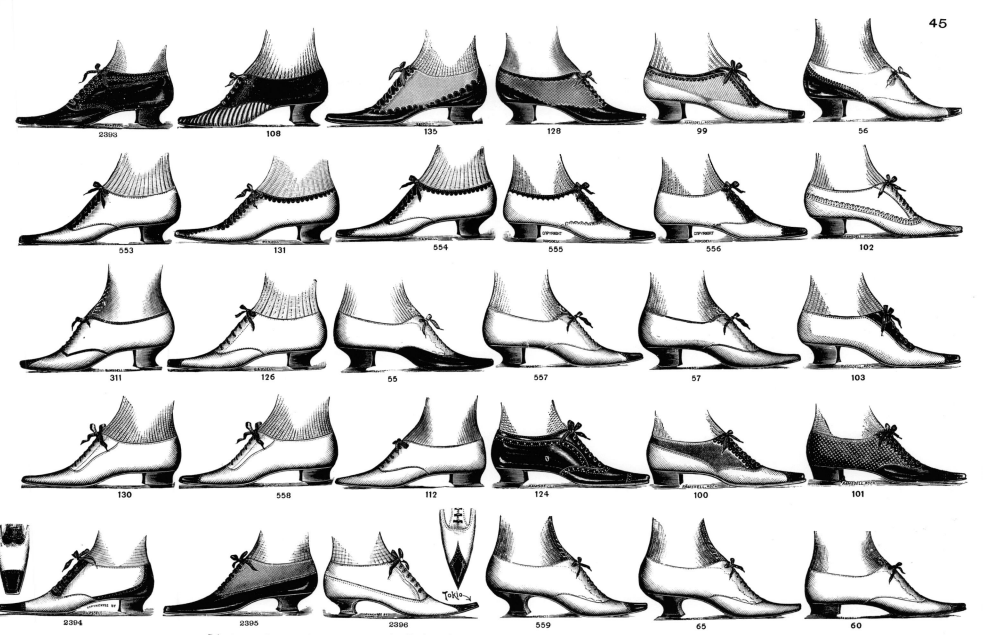

45

2393   108   135   128   99   56

553   131   554   555   556   102

311   126   55   557   57   103

130   558   112   124   100   101

2394   2395   2396   559   65   60

Price $1.00 each ; extra electros, 20 cents each.   Don't cut them out.

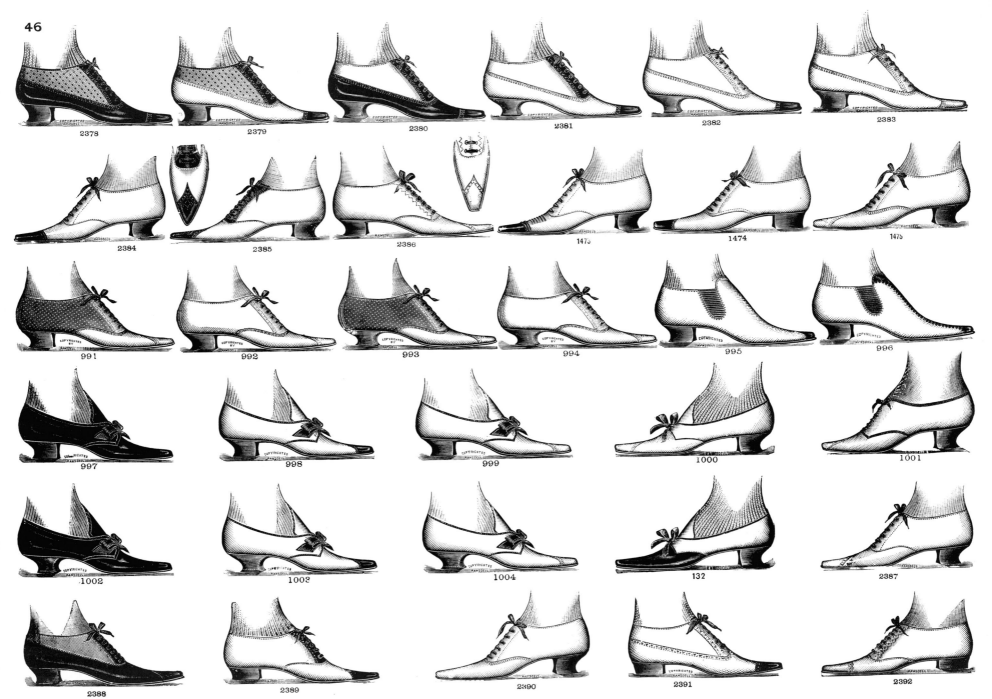

2378  2379  2380  2381  2382  2383

2384  2385  2386  1473  1474  1475

991  992  993  994  995  996

997  998  999  1000  1001

1002  1003  1004  132  2387

2388  2389  2390  2391  2392

PRICE, $1.00 each. Extra Electros, 20 cents.

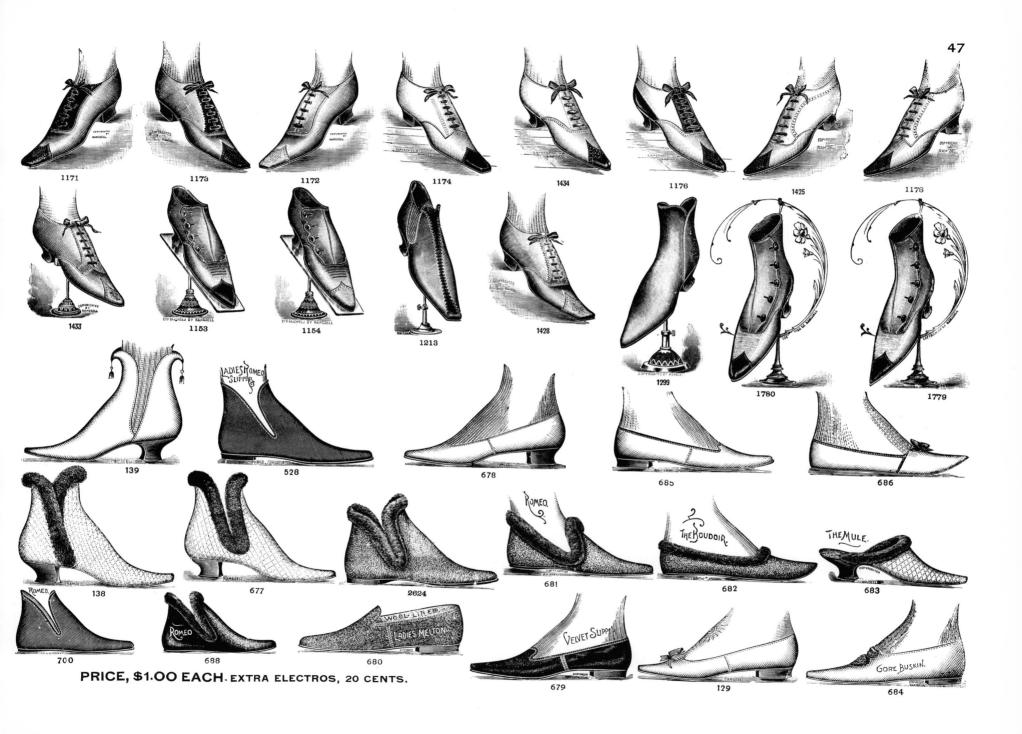

47

1171  1173  1172  1174  1434  1176  1425  1178

1433  1153  1154  1213  1428  1299  1780  1779

139  528  678  685  686

138  677  2624  681  682  683

700  688  680  679  129  684

**PRICE, $1.00 EACH. EXTRA ELECTROS, 20 CENTS.**

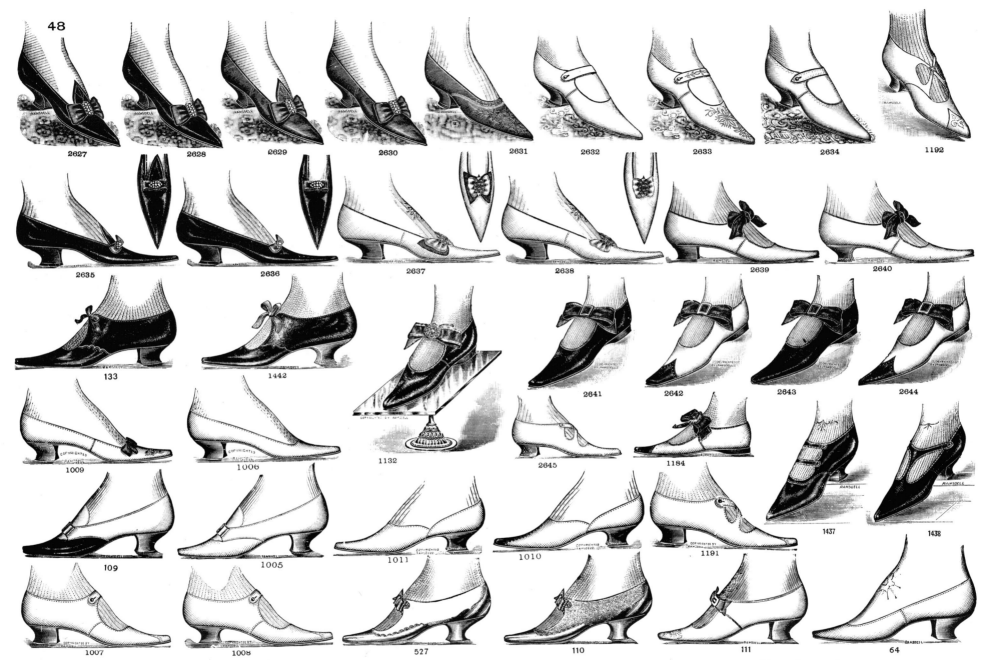

48

2627    2628    2629    2630    2631    2632    2633    2634    1192

2635    2636    2637    2638    2639    2640

133    1442    1132    2641    2642    2643    2644

1009    1006    2645    1184    1437    1438

109    1005    1011    1010    1191

1007    1008    527    110    111    64

**PRICE, $1.00 EACH.** EXTRA ELECTROS, 20 CENTS.    Your name cut in black places for 50 cents; in white places, $1.00.

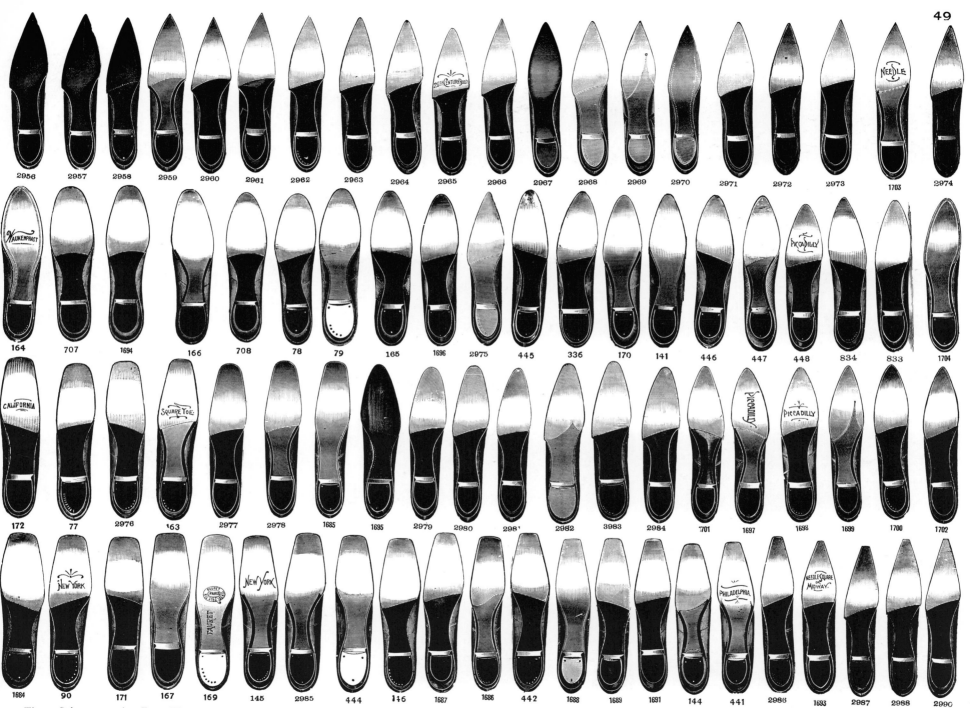

49

These Soles 5oc. each.    Extra Electros, 2oc.    You can order them put on  any Ladies' Shoe.    I will take out lettering on sole if ordered to.    If you order extra  lettering on soles it will cost you
50 cents each for  the first one of a kind.

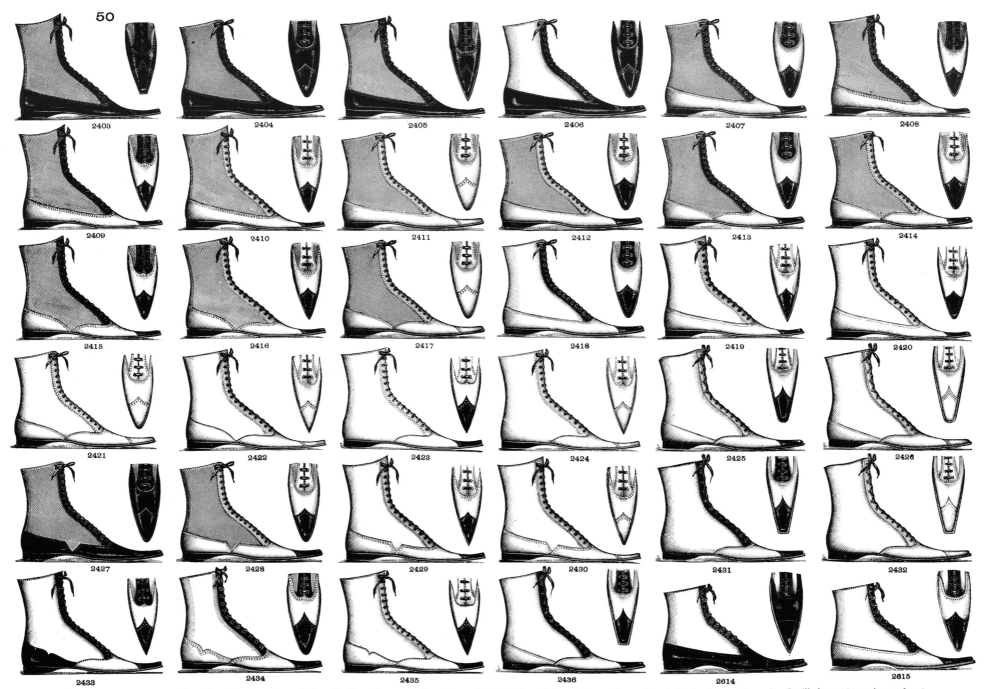

2403  2404  2405  2406  2407  2408
2409  2410  2411  2412  2413  2414
2415  2416  2417  2418  2419  2420
2421  2422  2423  2424  2425  2426
2427  2428  2429  2430  2431  2432
2433  2434  2435  2436  2614  2615

These Shoes cost $1.00 each without the front toes.   When the Front toes are left on they cost $1.50 each.   Extra electros with or without the front toes, 20c. each.   I will change toes when ordered.

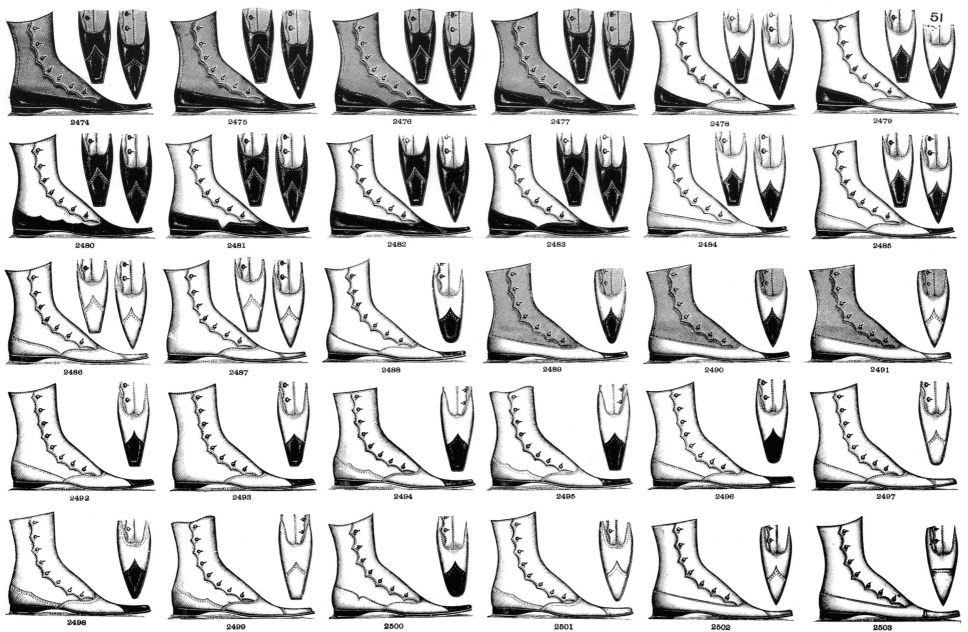

51

These Shoes cost $1.00 each without the front toes.    When the Front toes are left on they cost $1.50 each.    Extra electros with or without the front toes, 20c. each.    I will change toes when ordered.

52

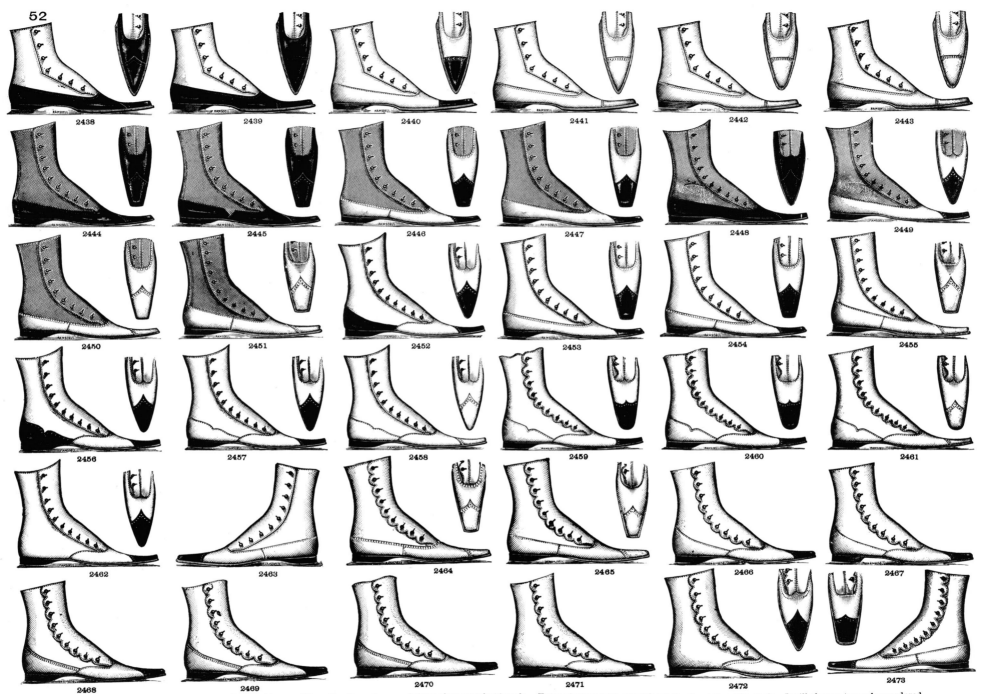

These Shoes cost $1 00 each without the front toes.    When the Front toes are left on they cost $1.50 each.    Extra electros with or without the front toes, 20c. each.    I will change toes when ordered.

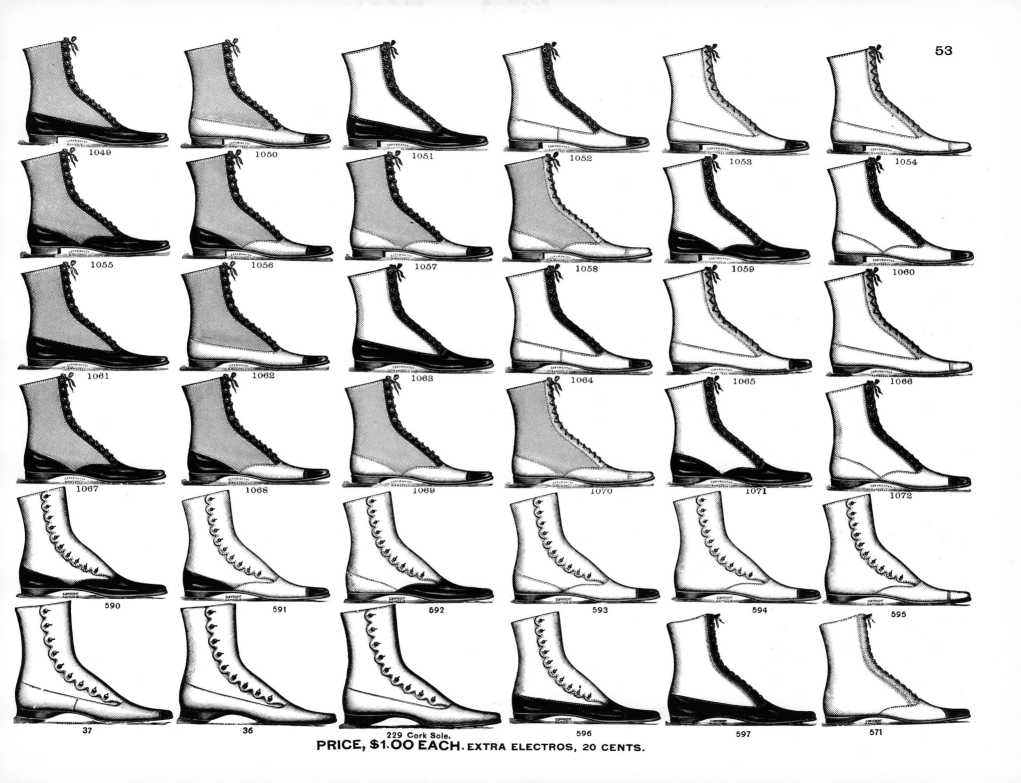

1049  1050  1051  1052  1053  1054

1055  1056  1057  1058  1059  1060

1061  1062  1063  1064  1065  1066

1067  1068  1069  1070  1071  1072

590  591  592  593  594  595

37  36  596  597  571

229 Cork Sole.
**PRICE, $1.00 EACH.** EXTRA ELECTROS, 20 CENTS.

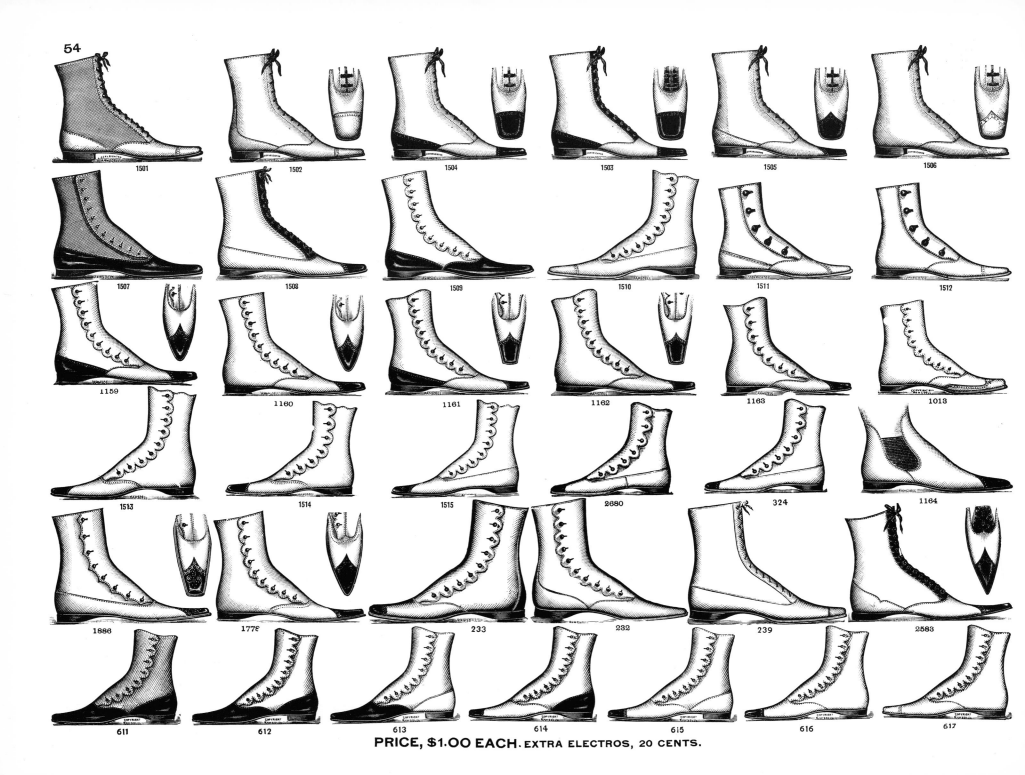

54

1501 1502 1504 1503 1505 1506

1507 1508 1509 1510 1511 1512

1159 1160 1161 1162 1163 1013

1513 1514 1515 2680 324 1164

1886 1778 233 232 239 2583

611 612 613 614 615 616 617

PRICE, $1.00 EACH. EXTRA ELECTROS, 20 CENTS.

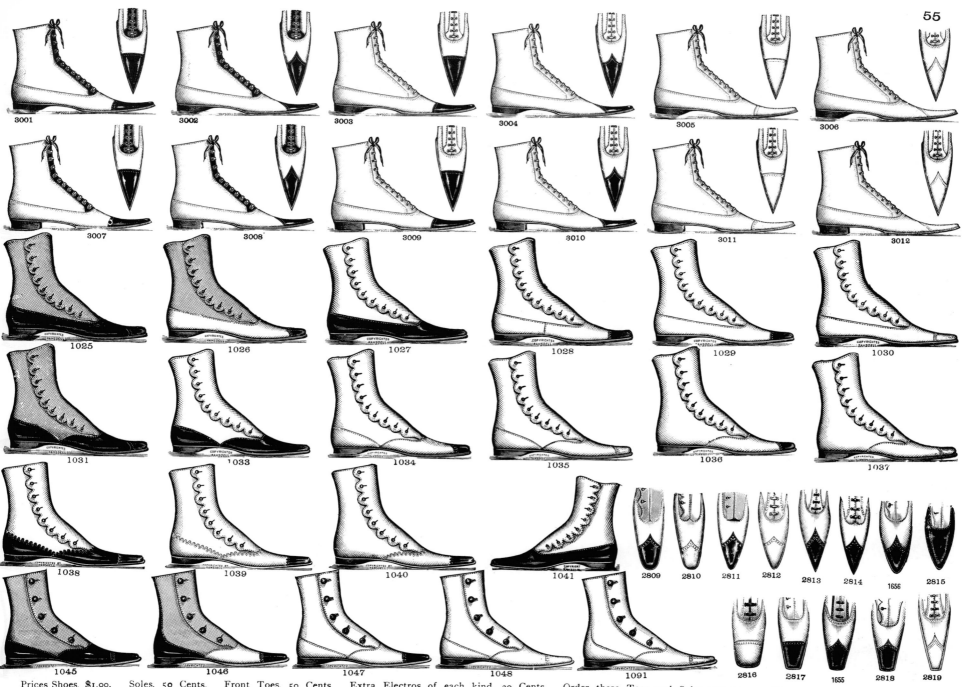

3001 3002 3003 3004 3005 3006

3007 3008 3009 3010 3011 3012

1025 1026 1027 1028 1029 1030

1031 1033 1034 1035 1036 1037

1038 1039 1040 1041

2809 2810 2811 2812 2813 2814 1656 2815

1045 1046 1047 1048 1091

2816 2817 1655 2818 2819

Prices Shoes, $1.00.    Soles, 50 Cents.    Front Toes, 50 Cents.    Extra Electros of each kind, 20 Cents.    Order these Toes and Soles put on any Shoes you want.

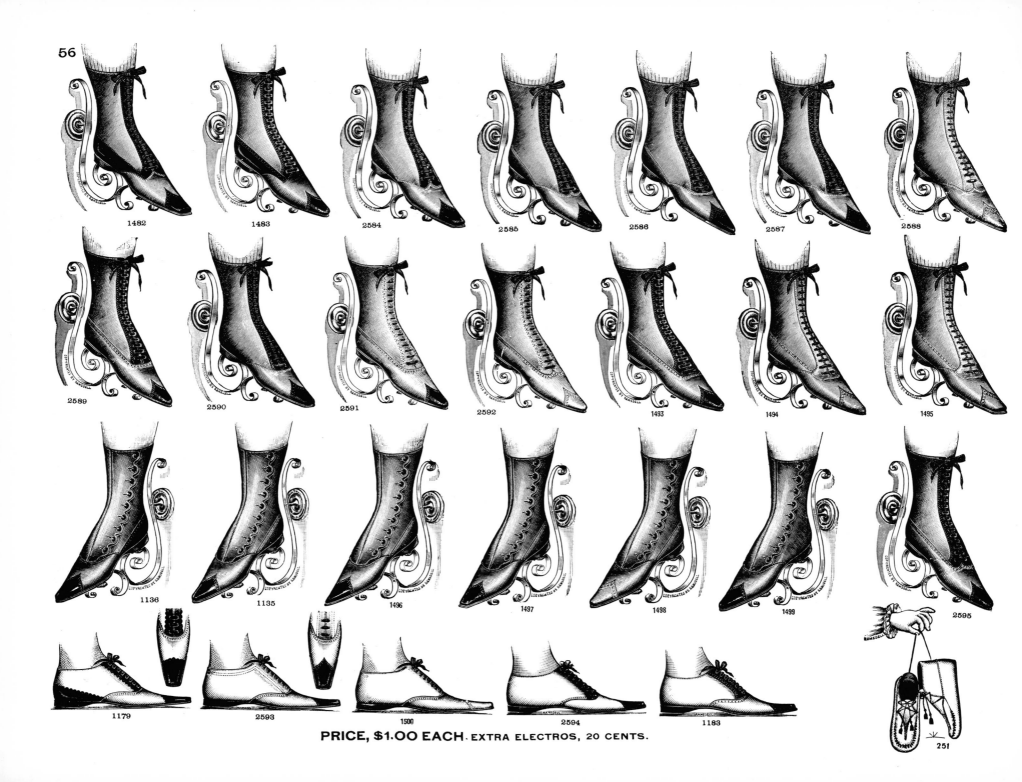

1482    1483    2584    2585    2586    2587    2588

2589    2590    2591    2592    1493    1494    1495

1136    1135    1496    1497    1498    1499    2595

1179    2593    1500    2594    1183

**PRICE, $1.00 EACH.** EXTRA ELECTROS, 20 CENTS.

251

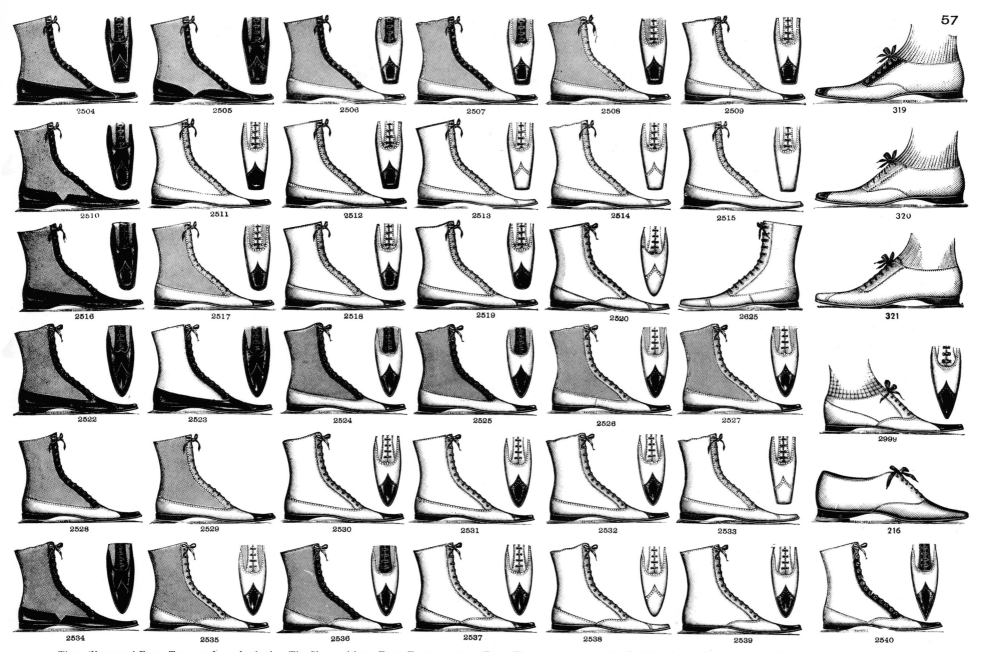

57

2504  2505  2506  2507  2508  2509  319

2510  2511  2512  2513  2514  2515  320

2516  2517  2518  2519  2520  2625  321

2522  2523  2524  2525  2526  2527  2999

2528  2529  2530  2531  2532  2533  216

2534  2535  2536  2537  2538  2539  2540

These Shoes and Front Toes are $1.00 for both.  The Shoes without Front Toes 75 cents.  Extra Electros 20 cents each.  I will exchange Toes from one Shoe to another when so ordered.

58

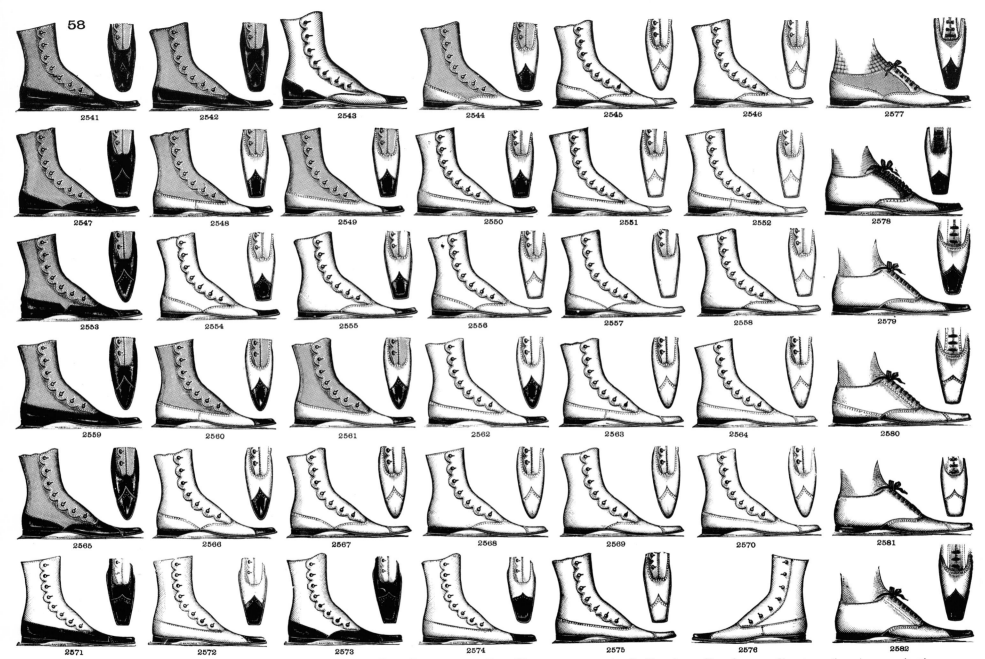

These Shoes and Front Toes are $1.00 for both.   The Shoes without Front Toes 75 cents.   Extra Electros 20 cents each.   I will exchange Toes from one Shoe to another when so ordered.

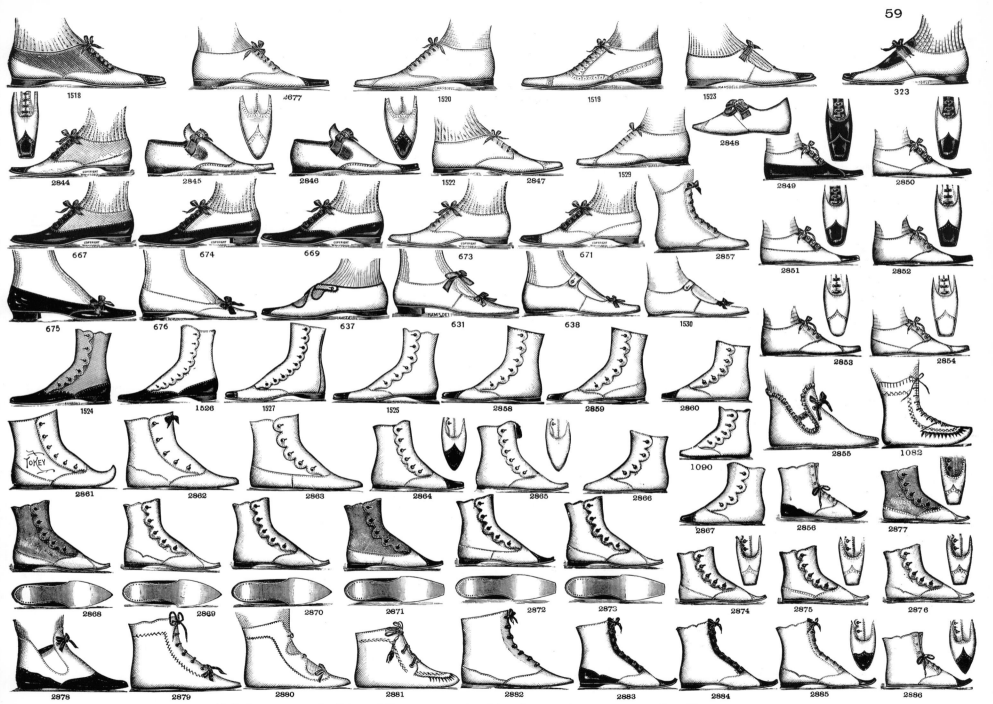

All Cacks, 50 cents each.   Soles and Tips, 25 cents each.   Other Shoes on this page, 75 cents.   Extra Electros, 20 cents.

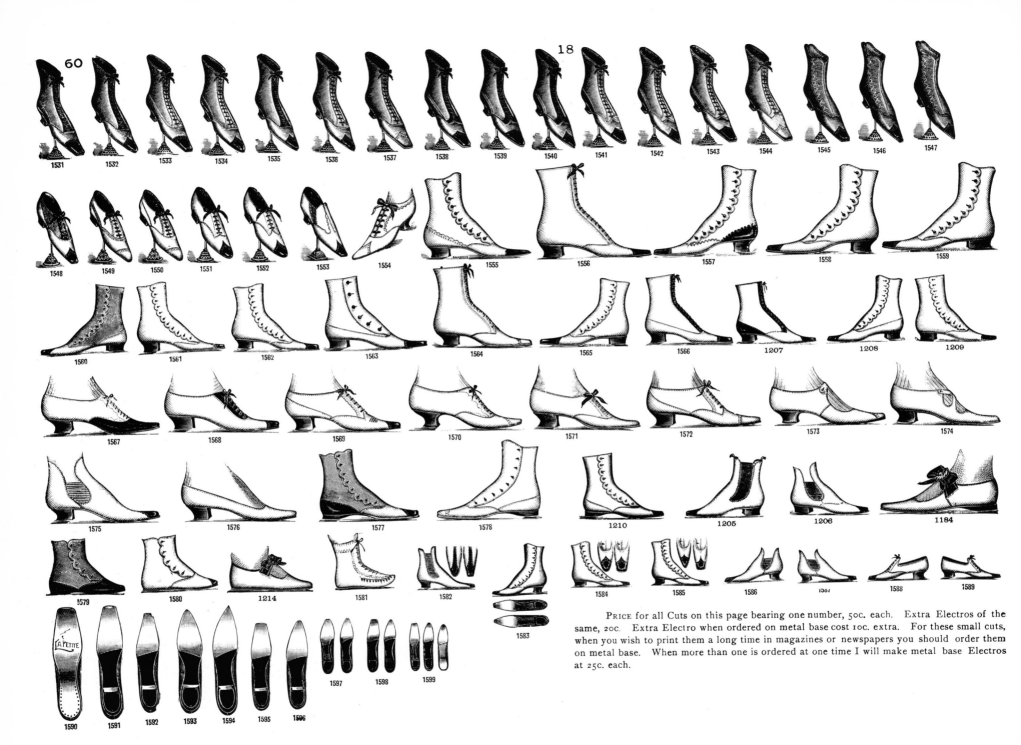

1531 1532 1533 1534 1535 1536 1537 1538 1539 1540 1541 1542 1543 1544 1545 1546 1547

1548 1549 1550 1551 1552 1553 1554 1555 1556 1557 1558 1559

1560 1561 1562 1563 1564 1565 1566 1207 1208 1209

1567 1568 1569 1570 1571 1572 1573 1574

1575 1576 1577 1578 1210 1205 1206 1184

1579 1580 1214 1581 1582 1584 1585 1586 1587 1588 1589

1583

LA PETITE

1590 1591 1592 1593 1594 1595 1596 1597 1598 1599

PRICE for all Cuts on this page bearing one number, 50c. each. Extra Electros of the same, 20c. Extra Electro when ordered on metal base cost 10c. extra. For these small cuts, when you wish to print them a long time in magazines or newspapers you should order them on metal base. When more than one is ordered at one time I will make metal base Electros at 25c. each.

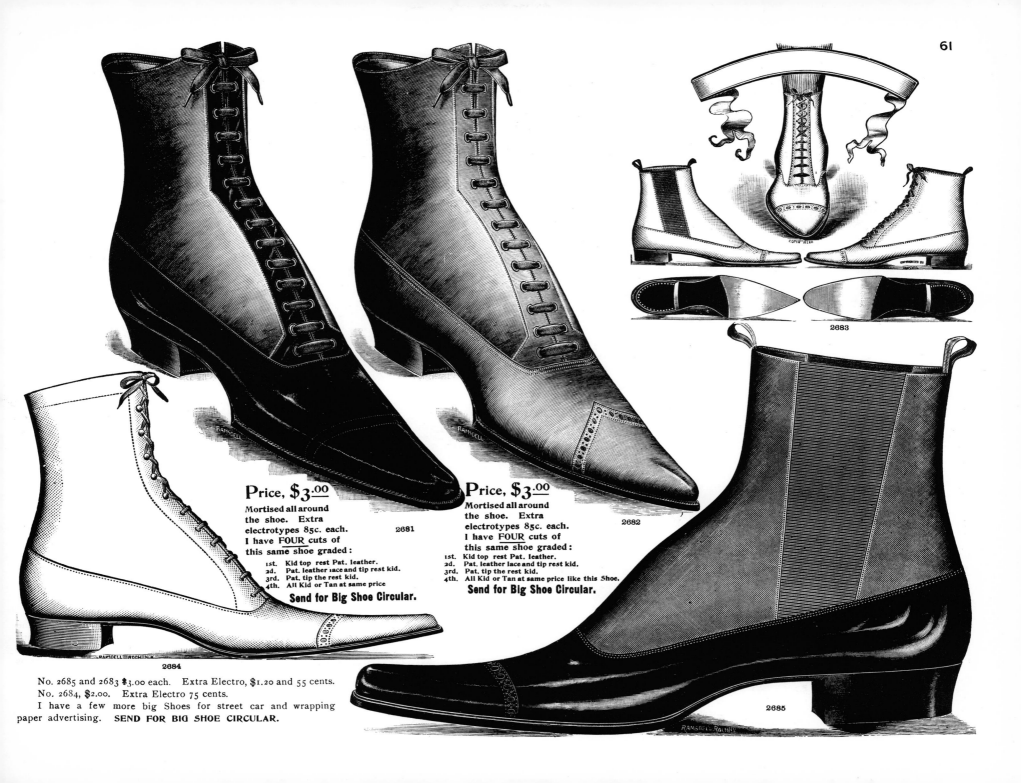

61

**Price, $3.00**

Mortised all around
the shoe. Extra
electrotypes 85c. each.    2681
I have FOUR cuts of
this same shoe graded :

1st.   Kid top rest Pat. leather.
2d.   Pat. leather lace and tip rest kid.
3rd.   Pat. tip the rest kid.
4th.   All Kid or Tan at same price

**Send for Big Shoe Circular.**

**Price, $3.00**

Mortised all around
the shoe. Extra
electrotypes 85c. each.    2682
I have FOUR cuts of
this same shoe graded :

1st.   Kid top rest Pat. leather.
2d.   Pat. leather lace and tip rest kid.
3rd.   Pat. tip the rest kid.
4th.   All Kid or Tan at same price like this Shoe.

**Send for Big Shoe Circular.**

2684

No. 2685 and 2683 $3.00 each.    Extra Electro, $1.20 and 55 cents.
No. 2684, $2.00.    Extra Electro 75 cents.
I have a few more big Shoes for street car and wrapping
paper advertising.   **SEND FOR BIG SHOE CIRCULAR.**

2683

2685

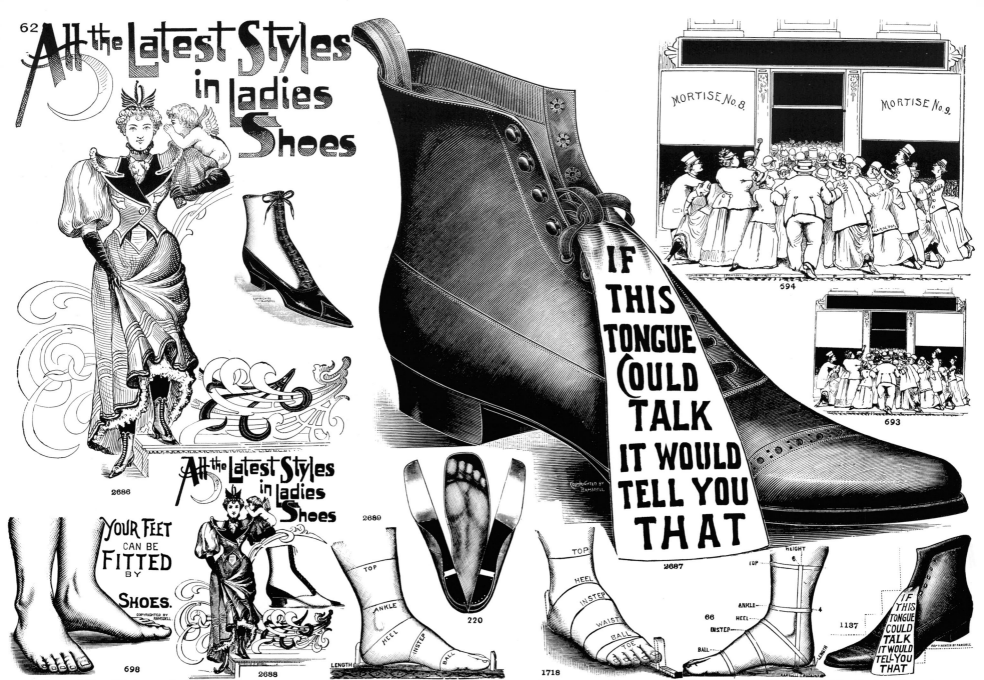

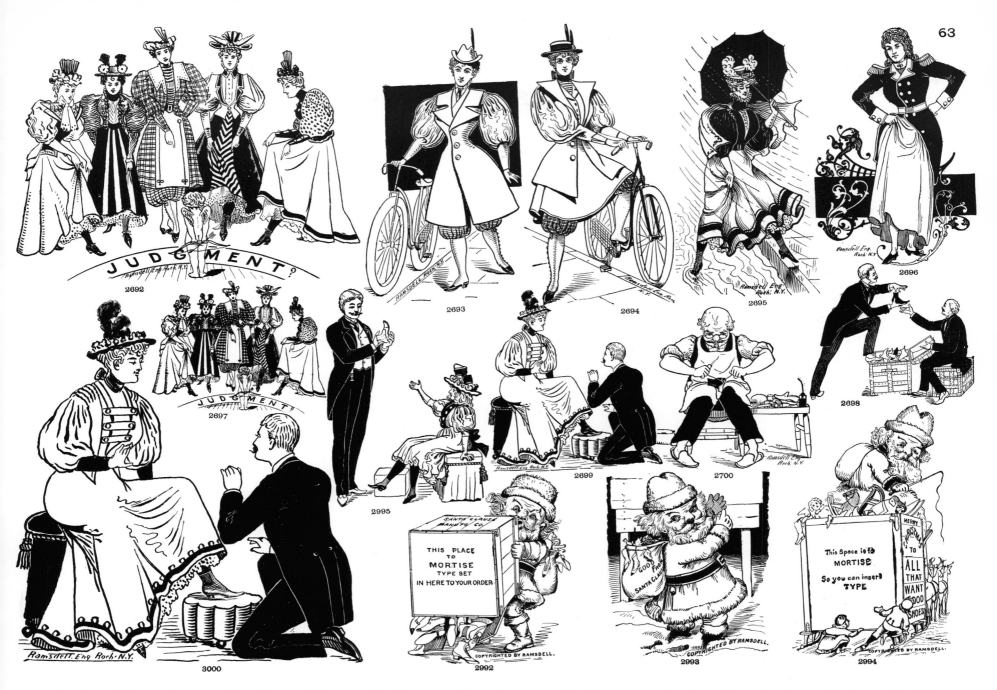

No. 2692 and No. 3000, $2.00 each.    Extra Electros of either, 75c.    All other cuts on this page $1.00 each.    Extra Electros 30c. each.    N. B.—I have all of these small cuts, especially the Santa Claus, in double column width, 4½ inches, at $2.00 each.

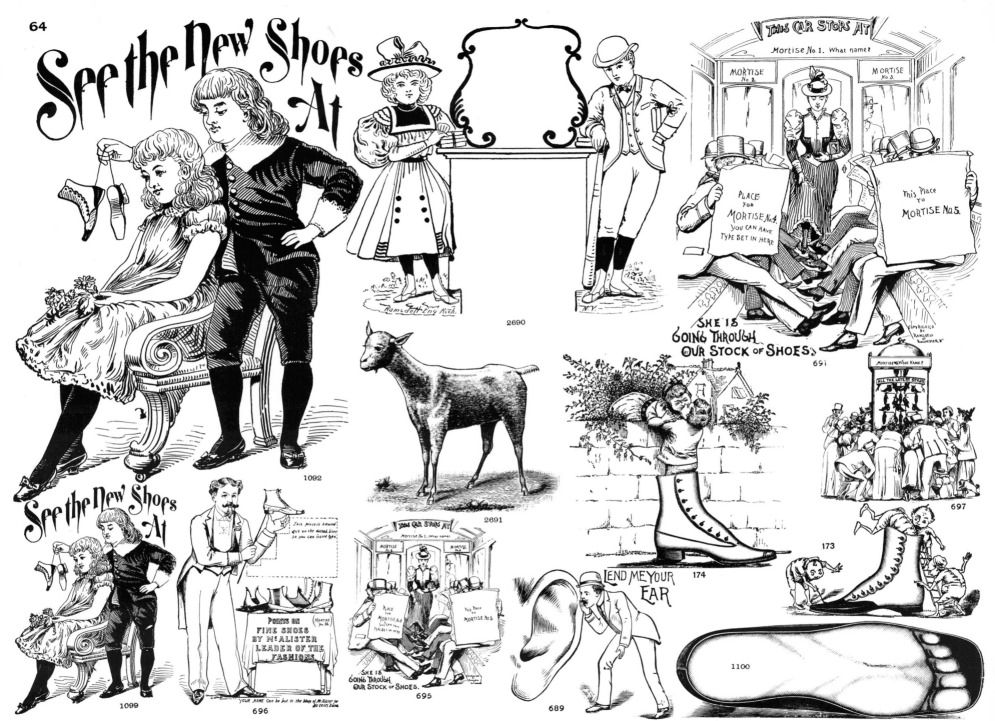